FITNESS
FOR HACKERS

code, lift, repeat
written by RYAN KULP

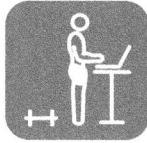

BONUS TOOLS AND RESOURCES

For additional tools and resources, book updates,
new case studies, and more, head over to:
fitnessforhackers.com

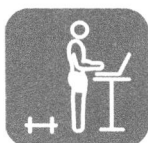

FOREWORD

You picked up this book because you're motivated to make a change and invest in your health. Let's get to the point: there's a lot of "lose weight, get fit" content out there and you'd like to know if the plan in this book actually... works.

As Ryan's wife, I'm uniquely qualified to confirm: yes, he followed the diet and workouts this book to the letter. No more and no less.

But we've all heard crazy weight-loss transformation stories. Ryan's story is among them. But why should you invest your time in this book?

#1: THE ABSENCE OF MAGIC

There is no magic bullet to reach your fitness or aesthetic goals. I recommend you avoid pills, infomercials and other hoopla that sing the tune of "lose weight without working for it."

Losing weight and gaining muscle are accomplished by two drivers. The first is a healthy diet and the second is a consistent exercise routine. There are no shortcuts.

Before reading, sit for a moment and mentally prepare yourself for the hard work. The good news is you're qualified to take on a challenge like this — you had the discipline to learn how to code. More people have figured out how to lose weight than how to code.

This book is a no-nonsense plan to learn 1 more skill that will literally extend your lifespan.

#2: SUITED FOR THE ACTIVE-AVERSE

I was a nationally ranked tennis player. From elementary school through college, I trained several hours per day. A strict training schedule included hours of weight-lifting, cardio, and tennis every day — sometimes one day off per week for "active rest."

While I'm no longer as hardcore as I was back then, I do not feel "myself" unless I exercise every day. Sometimes this means I sleep less or book gym time during a lunch or dinner break.

Ryan and I are opposites in this regard. I prefer additional gym time and do not have a restrictive diet. Ryan limits his workouts to a 30 minutes 3 times per week and restricts his diet.

When `Weight Loss = f(diet, exercise)`, you get some choice.

Yes, the right balance of diet and exercise may be different for you. This book is more suited for those who want a balance and aren't thrilled by exercise.

Ryan offers a few options in this book. Rather than get stuck in analysis paralysis because you're not sure what's right for you, just pick one routine and stick to it for 90 days.

#3: PROPAGANDA-LESS

Your favorite Instagram fitness feeds post pictures with hamburgers and milkshakes. You rationalize you'll just never look like them because even looking at hamburgers and milkshakes makes you fatter.

But what happens next? Possibly, the model spits out that comically large bite of hamburger, calls the end of the photo shoot, and heads to the gym.

Rather than feed you the highlights, Ryan covers each step he took on his weight loss journey.

Ryan does not have a good metabolism. In fact, Ryan used to be overweight. Ryan does not spend thousands on personal trainers. Ryan does not pretend to eat cakes and croissants. And, like you, Ryan has a demanding work schedule and cannot allocate much time towards his health.

This is the straightforward diary of what one "normal" guy did to get fit.

FINAL THOUGHTS

You've put in hours hunched over a computer. You've pulled all-nighters for hackathons or to patch a bug for a deadline. You've prioritized work or friends over your health. And now it shows. Because no one is going to invest in your health, but you.

Get ready to shift your mindset from labeling a special diet or gym time as selfish or indulgent behavior. You'll be a better employee, founder, husband, wife, boyfriend, girlfriend, or parent when you've taken care of yourself first.

Hideko Kulp

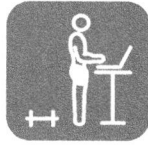

PREFACE

The last thing our world needs is another fitness book.

I wrote one anyway because no one has stepped up to serve my tribe, Hackers:

- software programmers who might not enjoy sports and physical activity
- ambitious professionals with little spare time for lifestyle-disruptive regimens
- those who value experiences over stuff, thus are more likely to binge eat, watch, drink, and do other activities counterproductive to good health

Anyone who reads this book, applies its principles for at least 90 days, and sends me a before/after progress pic, will get a 100% refund on the purchase price at fitnessforhackers.com/refund.

I'm not doing this to make money, I'm doing it to make hackers fit.

README.md
I am not an athlete.

For some, this is disqualifying information. I think it makes me a great candidate to share how you can become your best self. I also don't enjoy sports, running, hiking, or skiing, but I'm in better shape than a lot of former college athletes.

Besides feeling good and "being healthy," a few lesser talked about benefits of being fit:

- look great naked
- less likely to experience depression
- an edge in your career (recruiters/investors subconsciously trust and favor beauty)
- more Instagram followers
- outlive your college athlete friends
- less likely to get mugged
- more proactive in dealing with life's challenges
- an increased ability to focus on difficult tasks

Before we dig into workout plans, nutrition, mindset, and troubleshooting, here's my personal story. Consider it the paradigm of this book's data model. (*reminder: this is a book for hackers.*)

90S KID

I was born in the suburbs of Atlanta, GA. My father was a good athlete; my mom... not so much. My genes are slanted toward my mom, while my younger brother Kevin followed my dad's footsteps.

This means, growing up, I was the "chubby" one who got fat just looking at a Coke. Kevin could eat whatever he wanted. At some point, he took advantage of this, routinely offering me the last bit of his ice cream after dinner, which meant I then had to clean his dish. So maybe I did get my father's intellect (sorry dad).

While I never liked sports, I participated to make friends. I played baseball for 6 or 7 seasons, soccer for 1, tennis for 4-5, and even wrestling (freshman year of high school), and track & field (sophomore year of high school, though I never ran in a race).

In the back of my head, I knew being 'active' was good, even if I wasn't good at it. From pickup football games to skateboard and weightlifting, I experimented with a lot of physical activities growing up.

But I was always overweight.

GUT CHECK

My preferred definition of *overweight* is "weighing 20% or more above your ideal body weight."

So if you want to weigh 180 pounds but you're 216+, you are overweight. You don't need a DXA scan or finger blood pricks and definitely not a doctor to tell you this. Barring those exceptions of eating disorders, if you don't like how you look with your shirt off, you are also overweight.

My preferred definition of *obese* is when it hurts to look at yourself in photos, even with clothes *on*.

I was once obese in this sense. At 5 foot 11 inches, I weighed 240lbs and couldn't fit into any of the clothes I purchased only months prior. Making matters worse, my girlfriend and I had just filmed a funny video that went viral on YouTube, and it wasn't until I watched it that I realized how much I hated my appearance. It was time for a change.

YOUNG CAPITALIST

A few months after seeing my fat self on the silver screen, I moved to Harlem, New York City. Living 100 yards from 5th Avenue meant easy access to Central Park, so I bought a pair of Nike's and started running.

My route began at 105th street inside the Conservatory Garden. After 20 blocks southbound on the cobblestone 5th avenue sidewalk, I'd cut back into the park and work my way around the famous Jacqueline Kennedy reservoir.

At this point, runners are surrounded by tourists pouring out of the MET at 81st street, so my route home was northbound alongside Central Park West, on the park's interior 2 lane road for cyclists and service vehicles. Finally, I completed a half-lap around the Harlem Meer pond that opened up directly to my apartment's front door.

Running sucks. Especially when you're carrying around extra weight. But pain hurts a tiny bit less with a good view.

My weight began to shed, and it became an addiction: the scale read 220lbs, then 210lbs, then less—I lost 36 pounds by Spring 2013. I was pumped about my progress and started making protein shakes with my roommate's Vitamix.

Then my girlfriend cheated on me.

We broke up, and I started running longer distances, completing my first race (Brooklyn Half Marathon), then my second (Bronx 10k), then a handful of personal bests at the gym. Breakups are a leading marketing strategy for fitness club memberships.

So I started dating new girls. I went shopping for tighter clothes. Eventually, I settled on a woman who became my wife.

As such, the "break up, get fit" energy wore off. It always does, even if you don't find a new mate. So I reasoned with myself, *she wouldn't leave me for gaining a few pounds, right?* This is a selfish mindset, of course. Our partners in life—friends, spouses, even parents—deserve our best selves. We do too.

The next 5 years of my life were a series of more heavyweight fluctuations. They didn't all start with a YouTube video or end with a breakup, but what they did have in common was a pattern of conflict between the temporal and permanent.

- *temporal* motivations to work out → "aha" moments like a breakup, meditation, or unflattering photo
- *permanent* killers of temporal motivation → inability to control expectations, delay gratification, or measure results

It only took me all of my 20s to figure this out, but after 10 years of experimentation, research, and introspection, I finally embraced the new reality. Here it is:

If you want to be in great shape, avoid preventable illness, look good naked—all that jazz, you have to put your body under stress and control your eating.

Fitness is not, and will never be, a "kick" we can ride a few months and then forget about. I only lived along Central Park for 1 year. Then I spent 5 more years in New York City and visited the park maybe 20 times.

I only had a couple bad breakups to energize me into action, then I found the right person. I only had a job that let me off the hook at 5 o'clock for a couple years, then I became an always-on entrepreneur. Fitness is incongruent with the temporal, it requires permanence. You're reading this book because you already know this.

To reiterate, common sources of fitness kicks include:

- breakups
- upcoming special event (wedding, speech)
- seeing yourself in photos with better-looking people
- watching a YouTube time-lapse of a formerly fat person (*it's OK we've all been there...*)

If you catch yourself in the act of reacting to a fitness kick instead of acting out of a decision to be a better you, it won't work. You won't always have a wedding or photoshoot to design goals and deadlines around. You need something bigger to keep you going: you need to embrace the new reality (stated above) and believe there is no other way worth living.

A couple of years after my Central Park running binge had passed and I was again up 20 pounds (around 205 total), I joined Equinox, a $200+ per month premium gym with pools, classes, and a locker room with showers. I figured paying enough for a gym to make it "hurt" would help, and for a while, it did.

I also liked seeing "streak" check-ins on my Foursquare app. I obsessed about weighing in on the gym scales, and then my way-too-expensive $250 home scale, to watch the numbers go down. But the numbers didn't always go down.

Maybe it was just water weight. Maybe, I had too much to eat for a few days. Maybe, I just needed to take a big poop! It didn't matter because I was focused on 1 metric: mass in pounds.

GOING PRO

You might have had a similar experience as me: working hard to get in shape, the scale stops showing results, and you give up.

That's why Fitness for Hackers will equip you with 5 key metrics that create a *composite picture* of your overall fitness assessment and help you make intelligent adjustments to your health variables at a granular level.

Here are those metrics:

1. feeding windows
2. macros
3. muscle strength
4. body composition
5. mass

1. FEEDING WINDOWS

This one is simple: when you eat each meal, and how many meals you eat, all on a daily basis. A specific amount of time between feeding windows can help you accelerate fitness goals and keep your mind clear for work, relaxation, and life.

2. MACROS

We're going to primarily plan around fat, carbohydrate, and protein intake. You can read another book about vitamins and omega oils. If you're like me, you already have, and that didn't make a difference to your health. We are also going to count calories. It's old school, yes, and it works.

3. MUSCLE STRENGTH

Again, let's sidestep advanced biochemistry interpretations. We'll measure muscle strength by the amount of a specific, controlled movement you can handle for a given number of repetitions at a certain amount of resistance (weight).

4. BODY COMPOSITION

The size of each of your ligaments and muscles. We'll track the circumference of a few key areas, including your thighs, neck, chest, belly, and biceps.

5. MASS

How much you weigh. Often the only metric tracked by amateurs on a fitness kick who give up before they achieve their potential.

As you can see, weight is just 1 component of your quality of fitness. It's also devious, as *it will go up sometimes, even when you're doing everything right*. Remember this. Write it on your mirror or next tramp stamp. Sometimes you will weigh-in, and everything will look worse. That's why we track 4 other metrics, which I'll explain in a bit.

Back to my story.

GYM FATIGUE

A few months after joining a fancy gym, I was living in a great apartment with a great career and supportive people in my life. I could walk to the gym in < 10 minutes and essentially had zero excuses to not become a beast. A "Conan," if you will.

Then I started slipping. Like clockwork, my "I'm finally going to walk down there" gym routine shrunk from 4 times per week, to 3x, then 1x. The nail on the coffin was usually something like "*I'm traveling / busy / stressed at work with a big project*" and boom: back to 0 workouts per week with a $200+ gym membership. Idiot.

Why did I do this to myself? Why did I do this to myself over and over for 5 years? And what finally changed my approach to fitness and health?

That's what this book is about.

In short, here's how I learned to stay in shape (sustainably) and even find enjoyment in the process:

1. fixing my **mindset**
2. having a **simple** diet and workout plan
3. spending as **little time** in the gym and creating **systems**
4. avoiding **toxic** people, activities, and interests

This author won't bore you with a contrived acronym or mnemonic device like *MSST,* but here's one to help you at least remember my name:

- **R**eady?
- **Y**ou
- **A**re
- **N**ow.

PREPARE FOR CHANGE

The following chapters tackle each of these concepts—mindset, simplicity, time, systems, and avoiding toxicity—as they relate to achieving your fitness potential and becoming your best self.

In Part I, I outline the philosophy behind the Fitness for Hackers program and help you determine a better diet. We also equip ourselves with a tech stack conducive to measuring the 5 metris described above: feeding windows, macros, muscle strength, body composition, and mass.

Part II is where we hit the gym, set benchmarks for your current strengths and weaknesses, and implement systems into our routine to ensure fitness becomes embedded in our lifestyle, not just our to-do list. If you're new to working out in a gym, don't worry, I'll explain everything you need to know in words, pictures, and videos.

Finally, Part III covers advanced techniques to see more results, faster, as well as long-term maintenance (remember: sustainable) strategies and trouble-shooting techniques to avoid quitting. Whatever you do, you cannot quit.

MY PROMISE TO YOU

A lot of books, pills, and online courses will promise you a miracle. Here's my obligatory rebuttal: there is no substitute for hard work and persistence.

That's what makes you a hacker. That's why I wrote this book for *you*. It's because I know you spent 1,000s of hours learning your craft, and the global economy is vying for your skills. Your Maslow's hierarchy is mostly met.

But your body has suffered. And you're sick of hiding behind intelligence as a substitute for looking great. You want to understand what it feels like to *enjoy* working at a standup desk. Let's do that together.

Even the titles of this book's 3 parts are categorized according to my expertise as a marketer and software developer:

- Part 1 - Onboarding
- Part 2 - Activation
- Part 3 - Retention

Brought to you by a founder, entrepreneur, and hater of treadmills, here's the world's first fitness roadmap for hackers.

PART I >

ONBOARDING

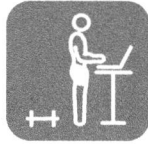

CHAPTER I

STANDUP MEETING

*"I used to play sports, then I realized
you can buy trophies."*
— Demetri Martin

Below are 4 ground rules to navigate this book and my point of view. I'll say these here, once, in classic DRY (don't repeat yourself) fashion. If you don't accept them, request a refund on Amazon.

NO BOOSTERS

I've read several books on health, tried 10+ brands of protein powder, watched 10s of hours of tutorial videos, and skimmed dozens of long-form landing pages about miracle vitamins and "superfoods" to figure out how others manage to stay fit.

A common denominator is supplements. These are usually in the form of pills, with excess metals, vitamins, and other chemicals that seek to enhance our "performance" (mental or physical) to gain more muscle or lose more weight faster.

While I'm not a doctor, I can safely share that supplements are not necessary to achieve a physique you're proud of. Also, they make life complicated as hell.

Imagine, in the midst of your busy schedule, setting calendar reminders to take XX milligrams of YY substance every ZZ hours, and some other thing every 3 days, then something else 45 minutes before a workout, and finally dissolving something else in your oatmeal at exactly 102 degrees but only on Tuesday or when it rains.

Supplements, while demonstrably effective for many people, are mental clutter. They take up valuable brainspace you probably can't afford as a knowledge worker, even if your wallet can. Since *simplicity* is one of our principles for sustainable fitness achievement, mental clutter is incongruent, and for that reason, **I will not recommend any supplements in this book**.

I do not personally take any supplements, and I'm in the best shape of my life.

FOR MEN

If you are a woman or you *identify* as a women, this book is not for you.

Women generally have different goals than men regarding body fat, tonality in their arms, areas of desired strength (e.g. hips), and so on. I've also observed that testosterone and men are being attacked by the media, so there are fewer places to learn and communicate with one another about male-specific challenges.

Assume from this paragraph forward that everything I'm saying is meant to be read by a man.

EXPERIMENTATION

You might want to read this book a few times. Not for my jokes, but to apply the concepts iteratively, just like in software and product development.

Fitness for Hackers is a 12-week program, but you'll learn in Part III that we can repeat the program again and again by increasing the difficulty.

Your MVP, or first program iteration, could be "stop eating X, starting doing Y." after seeing results, say 5lbs weight loss or 3lbs muscle gain, you'll prepare for version 2.0. Part of the human condition is challenging ourselves, after all. You do it at work, and now you can do it with your body.

Think of each idea I share as an experiment. You can try, embrace, reject, or refactor them into something better. Your body and diet are now a lab. The benefit of experimentation is that you never "fail" in a lab, you simply find another thing that doesn't work.[1]

KNOWING IS NOT ENOUGH

I won't wax poetic on different types of fats or omega oils. Why? Because nutrition textbook facts don't actually change our behavior. I read *Four Hour Body* just like everyone else and learned enough science to make my head spin. I was still fat, though, until I changed my *mindset.*

MINDSET IS EVERYTHING

In the following chapters, Fitness for Hackers explains exactly how to build, measure, and sustain strength gain as well as fat loss. Our leading principle as we progress, however, will be our attitude and mindset.

FAILURE IS INEVITABLE

Sometimes you write bugs in software. Probably every 20 minutes at work, and sometimes you will fail at your diet. You will fail your exercise plan. We will not allow failure to preclude success. Later in the book, I'll outline troubleshooting techniques to mitigate failure however you may encounter it.

SUMMARY

These are my ground rules for personal fitness. There are many like it, but these are mine.[2] now they're yours too.

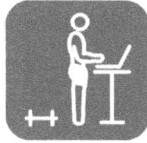

CHAPTER 2

CONFIGURING YOUR LOCAL ENVIRONMENT

"Worthless people live only to eat and drink;
people of worth eat and drink only to live."
— Socrates

It starts with what you eat.

I intentionally pushed "workout" concepts, specific exercises, and tracking tools to later chapters, because the path to being your best self, or at least having your best body, starts here.

Question: how often do you see a fat person at the gym who gets skinny over time? In my experience, they disappear. And the reason they stop working out often follows this sequence:

- people (my past self included) get fat by overeating and under-moving
- we eat to suppress stress, we eat to celebrate accomplishments
- anticipating a workout can induce stress (eat), finishing a workout induces pride (celebration - eat)

The last thing a health-seeking fat person should do is join a gym. Good health starts in the kitchen.

Following, are a few dietary frameworks to consider, each with their own challenges pending your relationship with food. Think of them like Rails, Laravel, Django; Alibaba vs. Oberlo; FIFO vs. LIFO; or whatever your favorite JavaScript stack is *right now*.

STANDARD AMERICAN DIET (SAD)

Jokingly referred to as the "seafood diet," as in *"see food, and I eat it,"* this is common fare for most people. There are no constraints or rules per se, just decisions driven in the moment by gut feelings. Want to "feel" healthy? Order a salad. Want to celebrate? Pizza. Notice your jeans are fitting too tight? Skip a couple meals or go for a long walk.

One cannot abide by the SAD to achieve fitness goals, this is merely included for reference. Pour one out for standard diets and standard people.

PALEO

Short for Paleolithic, a period of time often called the stone age or prehistoric era spanning 2+ million years, the paleo diet offers a simple heuristic: *could a caveman eat this*?

Allowed foods include fruit, nuts, lean meat, and fish. No, you cannot eat pure cane sugar. Many paleo followers do, however, consume natural sweeteners like honey or maple syrup. A lot of paleo food brands thus specialize in lightly sweetened snacks like cookies.

Paleo is similar to the "whole food diet" and is sometimes referred to as the hunter-gatherer or caveman diet.

KETOGENIC (KETO)

To illustrate the ketogenic diet *via negativa*, it's essentially the paleo diet minus carbohydrates, processed or otherwise. Some processed or modernized ingredients are OK in keto, but not paleo.

To get a better idea, for lunch, I usually eat:

- grilled chicken salad (lettuce optional)
- bacon cheeseburger (no bun)
- eggs, sausage, onions, peppers

and for dinner:

- pork chop, chicken breast (preferably skinless), steak (ribeye, filet, pending fat gram macro goals)
- a repeat of lunch but greater volume, e.g. triple bacon cheeseburger instead of a single patty

SLOW CARB

Coined by Tim Ferriss, this is a hybrid of paleo and keto. Certain carbs such as black beans are ok and cheat meals are also encouraged.

A cheat meal is when you follow your diet strictly for N days in a given period. Then, on the last day in that period, you eat whatever you want—your "cheat meal." Tim recommends 6 days "on," 1 day "off," with his personal choice being a blowout on Saturdays, candy bars and everything. Others will do 1 cheat "meal" per week instead of an entire day, reporting that a full day "off" can lead to feeling sluggish the following morning.

Since this book's goal and scope is to procure results within 60-90 days, I strongly advise against cheat meals until you've lost at least 10 lbs (if weight loss is your goal). If your goal is weight gain, have at it. We will turn that energy into muscle at the gym.

If you fear being unable to sustain a healthier diet without a little bit of cheating, try just once per month, or consider the Sweets section later in this chapter for a more frequent, less impactful style of cheating that won't reverse your progress.

CARNIVORE

Note: as of this book's publication, I follow the carnivore diet. While experimenting and writing this book, I was ketogenic.

Perhaps the newest entrant to the diet game, the carnivore diet is just as it sounds: meat only. Most folks who subscribe to this diet further restrict their meals to beef specifically, vs. a mixture of beef, chicken, fish, pork, or their neighbor's loud barking dog.

Extensive research is forthcoming, but a great resource to examine case studies outlining the benefits of a meat-only diet is meatheals.com, a crowd generated diary curated by fitness addict and licensed health professional Dr. Shawn Baker.

Many of the writers on Meat Heals have claimed that switching to a meat-only diet—even if their previous habits were also healthy (salads, reasonable calories, low sugar)—led to a reduction in diagnosed depression, joint pains, and inflammation.

I personally toggle between ketogenic and carnivorous eating styles on a per-meal basis. This explains my earlier lunch meal articulation of "chicken salad - lettuce optional." If I haven't pooped in a while, lettuce. If I'm fueling for a workout or replenishing my strength after a workout, I often go meat-only.

VEGETARIAN

This is the opposite of carnivore and equally as difficult to pull off.

While some vegetarians occasionally eat animal products like eggs, in general this diet is lower protein and higher in carbohydrates. Plant-based proteins like soy help vegetarians maintain and build strength.

PESCETARIAN

Vegetarians who eat fish regularly often identify as pescetarian. "Pesce" is the Italian word for "fish," and this diet is also sometimes called the Mediterranean diet for sharing characteristics of common meals in that region.

Animal products, including dairy and eggs, are also OK for many pescetarians. In general, pescetarians avoid chicken, beef, lamb, and pork but otherwise may follow a diet that looks similar to ketogenic, with more carbohydrates.

VEGAN

I don't have any "pros" for the vegan diet.

The word "vegan" was created by Donald Watson in 1944 while founding the Vegan Society. As an animal rights activist and pacifist, Donald was opposed to harming animals and thought veganism was *"vegetarian taken to its logical conclusion."*[3]

Only recently has veganism been compared with other diets as a contender for "better health," as its beginnings were based upon social and political sentiments about human ethics.

While veganism may indeed benefit the environment and slaughtering animals may indeed be inhumane, this is not a book about climate change or morality. We are focused on improving your body and mind, and animal products help on both counts.

If this rationale isn't good enough for you, let's make a deal:

1. get in great shape by consuming animal products and following the plan in this book
2. take a picture with your shirt off
3. switch to veganism for 6 months
4. take another picture and text it to me: 646.543.6458

If you look the same or better, I'll let you rewrite this section for a future edition of Fitness for Hackers.

LIQUIDS

After settling on our intake of solid foods, the other half of every diet is beverage.

I'll borrow sage wisdom from experts and simply say: avoid drinking calories. A few drinks that Big Food has lied to us about being healthy:

- orange juice
- really any kind of juice

I personally drink tap water, sparkling water, black coffee, and sometimes a little milk (dairy skim or almond OK) with the coffee if it's low quality. I also stopped casually drinking alcohol, but since it's one of my favorite hobbies I make exceptions for special occasions.

Here's my personal recipe for a quasi-iced cappuccino/vanilla latte. I call it a *prison latte*:

- almond milk or low-fat milk (or soy if you're soy)
- espresso
- vanilla extract
- (optional) sugar-free sweetener, e.g. Stevia

SWEETS

If you absolutely need sweet things in your life on a daily basis, explore fancy dark chocolates with at least 90% cacao. This is the "unsweetened" tier of chocolate, so it takes some getting used to, and I personally prefer eating just 1-2 squares at a time (< 100 calories) with a coffee in the evenings.

A quick glimpse at the difference in calories and macros between ~40 grams (a few small pieces, 1.4 ounces) of ordinary milk chocolate[4] vs. 90% dark[5] chocolate from Lindt:

	dark chocolate (90% cocoa)	milk chocolate	delta
calories	240	230	n/a
carbs (g)	12	24	200%
fat (g)	22	13	-41%
protein (g)	4	4	n/a
sugar (g)	3	22	633%

Dr. Brittanie Volk, a registered dietitian, says those on low-carb diets (including keto) should consume no more than 50g of sugar per day.[6] I think this number should be smaller, as consuming 50g likely means you're eating 2-3 sweet things that add up to hundreds of calories you don't need.

Sometimes, however, you'll eat sugar unintentionally. For example, you might order a grilled chicken dish, yet realize the "spicy" sauce on the side is actually "sweet and spicy" and thus has sugar in it. This recipe is a given for BBQ sauces and glazes (so don't order them!), but sugar is, unfortunately, a hidden ingredient in many prepared restaurant meals. Lesson: just be careful.

ARTIFICIAL SWEETENERS

Let's quickly settle the debate on adding sweeteners to your food and drinks. Some health purists claim that even "fake" sugar, such as the kind in a diet Coke, can have the same level of adverse effects on weight gain as real sugar.

This is partially true, and there's another option available for dieters with a sweet tooth.

Here is what you need to know:

- [real] sugar converts into glucose, which spikes your blood sugar and releases insulin
- insulin instructs your cells to absorb sugar from the blood, to reduce your blood sugar to a healthy level; this storage process causes fat gain
- [artificial] sugar, e.g. Sucralose or Aspartame found in diet sodas or powdered solutions like Splenda, does not convert into glucose but may "trick" your body into thinking blood sugar levels are high, thus inducing a release of insulin and increased fat storage

Leading research has found mixed results on blood sugar levels, and insulin release when using artificial sweeteners vs. sugar. For this reason, a personal diagnostic might be the best way to understand whether your body can "afford" to sustain sweet things in your diet.

For the rest of us, there is option #3, Stevia. Unlike aspartame and sucralose, Stevia is derived from a plant. Several studies have found that unlike other sugar substitutes, Stevia does not spike blood sugar or insulin levels, and is thus OK to consume by those on a fat-loss diet.

I asked Dr. Anthony Gustin, a certified sports chiropractor, functional medicine provider, and host of the Keto Answers Podcast, for his opinion on the matter:

> *"Stevia is one of the only natural sweeteners I recommend to my patients being as it comes directly from a plant. Not only does Stevia not have any negative health outcomes, it can actually improve insulin sensitivity and has been shown to have positive effects on gut health. There's no coincidence we use it for anyone trying to reduce the consumption of sugar, one of the most fattening things in the world."*

You can find Stevia at most health food stores and, increasingly, even some corner stores that sell coffee and other complimentary products. I usually "pinch shut" the same pouch of Stevia sweetener for 2-3 beverages over a 1-2 day period, further reducing my consumption to avoid any potential insulin spikes.

HEALTHY IS NOT ENTERTAINING

Restricting your intake to a few safe, repeatable meals might sound boring, so let's be honest: it is.

But this is also why it works… following a sensible diet means you don't salivate over your next meal. It frees us to adopt a mindset that food is fuel, not just entertainment. It keeps us satiated so we can focus on the Main Thing.

Right now, my main thing is running Fomo.com, learning how to be a good husband, reading books, and mentoring recipients of my scholarship program. A boozy brunch is incongruent with every single one of my daily, weekly, and life goals. A weekend of feeling sick (and regretful) is not worth 20 minutes of little chocolate cakes.

(a chocolate protein bar sweetened with Stevia provides 80% of the benefit anyway if you do need a pick-me-up.)

THE MOST IMPORTANT THING IS TO START

Whether you try a keto, slow carb, or carnivore lifestyle, you have to start now. Yes, you may have some leftover ice cream or salt and vinegar chips. Throw it all away and have a coffee to celebrate.

Get used to saying, "no bread please" / "no rice please " / "without the bun please" / "no potatoes, no toast." This will be painful at first, for two reasons:

1. not getting what you pay for feels like a huge waste of money (not all restaurants will take $$ off your bill)
2. bread, rice, potatoes, and black beans are amazing, but underneath the hood (your body), they convert to sugar and make you (or keep you) fat.

Some of you reading this can handle high amounts of carbohydrates in your diet: you are among the blessed few. This means you are insulin *sensitive*, whereas those of us (like me) who get fat just looking at a croissant, are insulin *resistant*.

If your goal is not to lose weight, and carbs don't turn you into an Oompa Loompa, you can throw this page of the book in the trash.

CARB FATIGUE

Everyone has a different relationship with carbohydrates. Excuses run the gamut of "my culture forces me to eat them" to "I'd die without them." none of this is true, but if it's what you believe, it's as good as law.

If you're primed to eating carbs every day—bread, potatoes, rice, beans, fleshy fruits like bananas—you'll probably feel fatigued and low energy after switching to a lower carb intake.

Pending your lifestyle and work schedule, you may want to reduce carb consumption over a 1-4 week period instead. The daily "recommended" carb count for a 2,000 calorie diet is 225-325 grams by BigFoodCo standards, and for reference, a slice of Wonderbread (white) is 14.5 grams.[7]

My personal goal as a keto follower is fewer than 30 grams of net carbs per day. I would aim for 0g, but as I mentioned earlier, it's normal for sauces, salad dressings, and even skim milk to have a few carbs here and there. I do not *ever* eat a slice of bread or rice. There will be plenty of time for baguettes in heaven.

To calculate net carbs, simply subtract the fiber and sugar alcohols from a food's total carbohydrate content. Leading low-carb protein bar provider Quest achieves this status with the following nutrition profile: 21g carbohydrates, 15g fiber, and 2g Erythritol. Health professionals debate "net" carbs as well as "good" and "bad" carbs. We are not so concerned. It is here Nassim Taleb reminds us, *"we do not need science to survive; we need to survive in order to do science."*

If you want to try this (remember, experimentation) but are carb-dependent, with sandwiches and pizza or chips as part of your regular intake, work backward over 4-6 weeks and reduce consumption from 350+ grams, to 250g, 150g, and so on until you reach a level that's tolerable and does not induce fatigue.

You may also replace carb-heavy items with low-carb alternatives as a stopgap to quitting carbs completely. One such solution this author used while trimming carbs from his diet was low-carb tortillas (4g net) as substitutes for bread. With these, you can make sandwiches, burritos, whatever. We'll talk about how to actually track your gram intake in the next section.

I confess that it took me several tries before I could "stomach" a full day without bread. But as Kate Moss says, '*Nothing tastes as good as skinny feels.*' You will stop craving pizza for breakfast. I promise.

SETTING A DIFFICULTY LEVEL

We often make the mistake of thinking a balanced diet means "balance of sugar, fat, and carbs."

Most people sort of just eat *whatever*. During lunch at work, you might get a salad to feel healthy, but on occasional Friday nights, you have a few drinks and crush a pizza.

Friends coming to town? Boozy brunch. Special event at work, or maybe a conference? Dinner rolls, beer, and those small dessert cakes. You can't help it—they don't serve healthy food at industry events!

Fortunately, today, you get to reject what's normal (obesity). But before choosing which dietary framework to experiment with, you need to set goals.

For most people just getting into, or *back* into, fitness, this means losing weight. For the lucky scrawny hackers out there, it means gaining muscle, widening your frame, or developing endurance and stamina.

Here are a few body types I collaborated with in writing this book. If you identify with one of them, this will help you figure out dieting and intensity levels to establish in the next section.

SKINNY FAT

Your body either doesn't gain weight easily, or you restrict calories to remain a certain size. You don't work out, but you look OK. Try to run a mile, however, and your lack of fitness is evident.

AVERAGE DEV

You don't have to build software to fit this mold. A lot of desk jockeys "suffer" from this degree of complacency: you look OK with your shirt on. In the past, you looked better, perhaps during a fitness kick or when you "used to play sports."

PLUS-SIZED

If this is you, I'm sorry. I tease fat people a few times in this book because fat-shaming… works. I used to be fat too. I was 235 pounds, 5 foot 11 inches, and did not have a gym membership. Search online for "ryan kulp Korean girls" to see how I carried that weight. I was begging to be mugged.

Plus-sized hackers are often successful professionally and therefore a) highly stressed or b) constantly celebrating. Either case leads to overeating. If you are never mistaken for a model, you might be plus-sized.

SETTING GOALS

Next is a simple compass to help determine which diet to try first, where "try" = 3+ months implementation with minimal (hopefully zero) deviation. If you prefer imagining an error logger being installed on your diet, you should have fewer than 2 critical bugs per week and no pager duty necessary.

GOAL: LOSE WEIGHT

Whether you want to lose 5lbs or 50lbs, the only way to hit your goal weight (and stay there) is to do so sustainably. Using the chart below, be honest about how your body responds to carbohydrates, then choose an intensity level underneath that feeling.

eating carbohydrates makes me feel...	bloated	sick	perfectly fine
I prefer a lower intensity program	slow carb	keto	avoid sugar, alcohol
I prefer a higher intensity program	keto	carnivore	slow carb with multiple cheat meals

For me, I feel sick if I eat too much bread, and I consider myself a high energy person.

Thus, my baseline diet is ketogenic with 1-2 deviations per week to carnivore. Buying meals a la carte at steakhouses is one way I practice the carnivore diet, eating 3-4 beef or chicken skewers for lunch is another. I find these at street carts and shopping mall food courts when I'm not eating salad to help me poop.

Takeaway: if your goal is to lose weight, assign yourself a number greater than 10 pounds (4.5kg). If you prefer to lose less than 10 pounds, you're probably seeking body composition changes.

GOAL: BODY COMPOSITION (CONVERT FAT TO MUSCLE)

Suppose you're a 6-foot tall man that weighs 190 pounds (86 kg). You haven't worked out much and identify as an Average Dev. Your body fat is somewhere between 18-28%,so it makes sense to swap out some of that fat for muscle.

Since it's difficult to do two things at once, I want you to follow the same diet as someone who needs to *lose* weight, then reconfigure your goals to *gaining* weight around the 3-month mark.

This means you'll spend a few months running a calorie deficit, optimizing for fat loss vs. muscle gain. Then you'll switch routines to de-emphasize calorie cuts and intensify your workouts to pack on more muscle, faster, while maintaining a comfortable, sub-10% level of body fat.

Takeaway: if your goal is improved body composition, take a lot of progress pictures and get professional scans for granular insights into your bone and muscle density. We'll discuss these scans later in Chapter 4.

GOAL: GAIN WEIGHT (FAT + MUSCLE)

First, I hate you. Just kidding. Sort of.

Your primary goal is simply to get stronger. As strength increases, so does body mass. As you build a body that needs more nutrients to self-maintain, you'll naturally begin to eat more without feeling sick.

If you like running, stop running. If you prefer doing lots of repetitions at the gym with smaller weights, stop doing that too. I'll explain exactly the type of workouts you need in Chapter 4, but in general, we are going to toughen up and intensify your diet and workout routine. We're going to make you bigger.

In the meantime, I suggest a moderate carb diet with 2-3 cheat meals per week. Substitute low-calorie proteins like chicken with high caloric and fattier proteins like pork. Eat fatty, marbleized ribeye steak vs sirloin. Buy sugar-free, organic almond butter and learn to drink milk. If you apply these modifications—along with our workouts in the coming chapters—and still don't lose weight, see a doctor.

Takeaway: if your goal is to gain weight, assign yourself a number between 5-20 pounds (2.25 - 9kg).

CALORIE COUNTING

Some fitness experts argue that it "*doesn't matter how many calories you eat, as long as you are eating the right things.*" I don't subscribe to this, and even if it worked for my own body, most of us physically feel *worse* if we overeat.

For me, this becomes apparent whenever I plan to hack on a side project after a big dinner. My stomach is busy hoarding blood flow to digest the food, leaving less bandwidth for my brain to get back into work mode and create things.

Just as a single glass of wine can greatly reduce your concentration (without increasing your level of entertainment), the composition of a meal can impact a knowledge worker's endurance. Even 200-300 more calories than necessary can create a fog that makes work unappetizing. Too much salt in a meal can lead to extreme sweets cravings, the old "going out for dessert" routine. And if an entire meal is served cold, you might want another one just to taste something hot.

All of this begs a myth-buster that cannot be overstated: humans do not naturally get tired of working after 5pm. It's simply that we stuff our bodies and are *incapable of complex thoughts after dinner*, so we resign ourselves to Netflix instead of becoming our best selves.

Whether calories should be counted or not is not the point: we are simply less productive when we overeat, so we'll count away. Here's a compass to establish an appropriate daily caloric intake, assuming your goal (like mine) is to lose weight:

goal weight	height (feet/inches, cm)	suggested daily calories
< 135	5' 0" - 5'6 (XX cm)	1500
< 165	5' 7" - 5' 11" (XX cm)	1750
< 185	6' 0" - 6' 2"	1900
< 215	6' 3" - Yao Ming	2,200+

I personally aim for fewer than 1,750 *net* calories per day, and I'm 5 feet 11 inches tall. OK, maybe 5 feet 10 inches and 3 quarters.

By *net,* I mean that I can consume closer to 1,900 calories if (and only if) I also walk at least 2 miles or have a hard 30-minute workout. Each mile walked burns about 100 calories, pending your weight, speed, terrain, and incline.[8]

If your ideal caloric intake seems low and eating is your favorite thing, counteract it with more activity. Just don't *celebrate* activity with food. We'll talk more about this later in Chapter 8.

SNACK STRATEGY

The first rule of Fight Club: don't snack.

Most "healthy" snacks got that branding because they are < 100 calories, which has nothing to do with ingredients. Further, processed foods that manage to pack < 100 calories usually have stuff in them you don't want in your body anyway.

Experimenting with a new diet usually introduces 2 pangs immediately: first, carb fatigue, which we discussed already. Next, "boredom" at night, between dinner and the time you go to bed.

I believe this window—the space between dinner and bedtime—is the Achilles heel of most diet plans and fitness regimens out there. Humans simply can't stop eating. And it's easy to crush 500+ calories every night without even looking at your hands, which is 1+ pounds per week you could otherwise be losing without a single workout. We'll address how to quash this nasty habit shortly when we introduce intermittent fasting.

A night owl myself, fixing my snacking habit was a lot more difficult than going without bread. It's normal for me to be on my computer, hacking or writing, until 2-4a every night. Even if I have a late (8p) dinner, this means

I have to last 5-7 more hours with nothing but water. And let's be honest, I drink coffee past dinner too.

After a few weeks of fumbling around, I identified 2 simple ways to avoid snacking at night:

- brush your teeth after dinner
- don't buy snacks

Similar to our 4-6 week carb reduction plan, you don't have to go Cold Turkey on snacking if it's become a staple part of your lifestyle. First, buy at least 1-2 fewer items on your next grocery run. If you're used to loading up 3-4 bags of chips, crackers, and 1 ice cream pint, skip the ice cream this week. You can trade 40+ evening hours of willpower at home if you practice 30 mins of self-control at the grocery store.

After a week or two of rationing your snack intake, institute a No Snack Saturday. I've found that waking up on Sunday not bloated or hungover is an optimal way to prepare my body and mind for the work week ahead.

Finally, find a liquid substitute for snacks. For me, this is sparkling water. Ever since La Croix made their comeback, I've been crushing 1-3 cans /night at home. Carbonated water can make you feel bloated, but it also fills you up, and the bloating will go away in the morning.[9]

FIND AND REPLACE

Here are a few alternatives you can `shift+cmd+f` in your diet to avoid going insane while easing into a new routine:

- coffee → non-dairy additives like coconut or almond milk, or simply a couple drops of vanilla extract + cinnamon
- pizza → just no. (*if you want to try the hipster cauliflower crust everyone in Oakland is talking about, be my guest*)

- sandwiches → "unwich" style, aka lettuce wrap instead of bread. Ordering this in front of friends / colleagues is actually kind of fun. They'll look at you sideways but secretly wish they had the nerve to do the same.
- Asian → no more sesame / general chicken / egg rolls. Thai and Japanese preferable vs. Chinese. Choose spicy > sweet (honey-based) sauces if you can handle the heat. No more gyoza, sorry.
- salads → even these can be improved, e.g. ask for "no croutons" and definitely no bread on the side. Some dressings are fatty, i.e. olive oil, but I personally don't censor my fat (grams) intake at all.

As you figure out your home life and personal meal schedule, each passing day will get a little easier as your stomach anticipates the new constraints. You might even see quick results (2-3 lbs lost) in as little as 7-10 days, simply by reducing your snacking and making each meal or coffee incrementally healthier.

FRIENDS

Our amygdala, sometimes called the lizard brain, is hard enough to conquer as we improve our food consumption. What's even more challenging are friends. Specifically, friends in better shape than us who seem to eat and drink whatever they want without impact.

The first thing to realize about this special group of people is that they might be *lying*. It's not uncommon for a gym rat to hit the bars—hard—on a Friday night. They just starve themselves on Saturday and run an extra 2 miles Sunday. They could also be "skinny fat" or wear an evenly distributed amount of fat on different parts of their body.

This realization hit me while reading Robert Greene's *48 Laws of Power*.[10] specifically, Law #30: "Make your accomplishments seem effortless."[9] for women, this helps explain some of those Instagram models sitting on a breezy beach balcony with a huge burger and fries in front of them. For men, think of frat guys at the bar with tank tops, tattoos, biceps, and Bud Light.

Yes, some people have a special metabolism. But no, you are not one of them, and neither are most people. I learned this the hard way (see: puking in Manhattan) that a couple hours of "enhanced" fun is never worth a terrible next day or even a regretful 20 minutes in bed, waiting to fall asleep while feeling bloated.

Let friends do their thing, and you do yours.

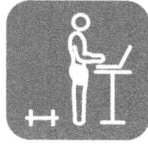

CHAPTER 3

QUANTIFIED SELF

*"If you eat lunch with your shirt
off, you'll eat less lunch."*
— Unknown

Before you can get fit, you have to decide what fit even means.

For most of us, this is pretty simple: "lose weight" or "gain muscle" or both. But hackers are more specific in their approach. Here are a couple example goals you might want to steal:

- lose 10 pounds in 60 days
- run a 5k in < 20 minutes (*6 min, 25 seconds per mile*) by this Summer
- finish the *Spartan* obstacle race and beat my friend Jeff

Whatever you choose, scope it to be achievable within 90 days. If your goal is ambitious, i.e. to lose 50 pounds, set sequential goals, and "unlock" them over time: 20lbs in 90 days, 15 pounds in 70 days, 10 pounds in 60 days, and the last 5 pounds in 6 weeks.

PICK A GOAL, ANY GOAL

Besides the great feeling we get after *achieving* a goal, *setting* goals keeps us grounded on the "bad" days. Earlier I broke the news that you absolutely will step on the scale sometimes and weight 5lbs more than you did a week ago. The human body is nuts, and progress is non-linear, just like startups.

Another reason you need to set a goal is so you can call BS on this book and demand a refund, or measure positive results and *earn* a refund. Either way, this book is free, so long as you follow it.

On bad days, goals are like a big hug from your partner. On good days, goals look like jokes, and you'll be tempted to reset them for something more ambitious.

I recommend setting a goal, achieving it, then looping the process again and again. If you constantly reset goals before reaching them, your psyche will suffer. Don't let your spirit miss out on the feeling of a checked box.

With your fitness goal in mind, make a copy of **this spreadsheet** *https://docs. google.com/spreadsheets/d/1w_2xgcEij1as7JK9-FEEwK4FsUaaCgEem9FQPM 5FdPM/edit#gid=0* and write it down in Cell B2.

Completing this step is what's known as an *Implementation Intention*, a term coined by psychologist Peter Gollwitzer.[11] in his research Gollwitzer found that a simple "If-Then" commitment strategy for desired behaviors increases the probability of that goal being accomplished.

So whether it feels silly or not, make a copy of the spreadsheet above and fill in the blanks as you continue reading.

TRACKING ALL THE THINGS

For 90 days, starting now, I want you to use this book and these free products to ensure hyper-awareness of your goals and thus increased assurance of their achievement.

- **Zero**, for intermittent fasting (iOS / Android)

- **Trello** for workout routines and gains
- **MyFitnessPal** (iOS / Android) or **LoseIt** (iOS / Android) for calories, macros, and progress pics
- **Google Sheets** (the template link above) for body and muscle sizing

ZERO

Intermittent fasting is restricting your body to 4, 6, or 8-hour "feeding windows" vs. the usual all day slaughter of snacks and meals. By doing this, in short, your metabolism speeds up, and your focus improves at work.

LAST 7 FASTS

Goal 16 hours

FRI	SAT	SUN	MON	TUE	WED	THU
1/25	1/26	1/27	1/28	1/29	1/30	1/31

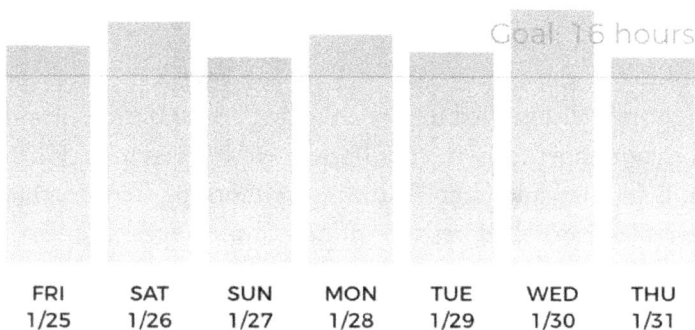

A few years ago, I fell in love with Chocolate Chip Cookie Dough Quest Bars, which is a 20g protein bar that has just 4g net carbs (total carbohydrates minus fiber).

I ate 1 every day for breakfast, along with a coffee and a book. But then I started eating them in the afternoon... on my computer after midnight... in the bathroom at my favorite restaurant (*just kidding, kind of*).

Quest Bars are great sources of protein, but they're also 190 calories /each. Since a pound represents 3,000 - 4,000 kilojoules, I missed out on potentially half a pound per week of weight loss just by eating 1 per day. Not to mention, eating a processed protein bar begets at least 1 beverage, as fibrous foods compel thirst.

Ultimately that accompanying breakfast coffee often had a bit of 1% milk (50 calories) and artificial sweetener (increases insulin resistance). For some of us, breakfast also has the tendency to "rev up" your system, and by 11am, you're already wishing it was lunchtime.

To join the #NoBreakfastClub and start fasting intermittently, go with the 16:8 sequence and start your time (Zero app) tonight after dinner. My schedule: dinner around 19:00, finished by 20:00, then not eating again until lunch (noon) the next day. At least a few times per week, I'm not even hungry until around 2p, and I can pull off 18-hour fasts from 20:00 - 14:00.

Skipping breakfast can assist in up to 1 pound a week in weight loss, but it does taking some getting used to. Try chugging 20-30 ounces of water to further reduce your appetite as you get started with this routine. Growing up, I had cereal, Pop-Tarts, and Eggo Waffles every morning (seriously), and in my early to mid-20s, I switched between protein shakes, eggs, and bacon.

While eggs are a big step up from Cinnamon Toast Crunch, the reality is I restricted my intake to 1,750 calories per day. Do I really want to wipe out a third of that by 9am? I'd much rather enjoy a steak later, with company after accomplishing something.

Zero provides a couple big buttons you can push to start or stop a fast, and it's easy to modify timestamps if you forgot to hit 'start' or 'finish' after the fact. Finally, Zero has an export option that we'll use in the spreadsheet you copied earlier.

I suggest you fast 16 hours at least 3 times per week.

TRELLO

This is our tool of choice for what happens in the gym. There are many, many fitness trackers and I've tried a lot of them. But we don't need push notifications, a social network, paid monthly subscriptions, or anything fancy to stay in great shape and visualize progress.

Here's a screenshot of my current workout routine. Note the "A" and "B" days with a third list for historical gains. In Chapter 5, we'll dig into each of these workouts and why you don't see more than 1 "set" per exercise in my regimen.

A-Day (back, chest, arms)	B-Day (legs, shoulders, traps)	Gains
Dips (36)	Curls (90x14)	Triceps press down (60x11)
Biceps curls (90x14 - bar)	Dips (31)	Bench or chest press (160x5, 150x10)
Bench or chest press (160x10)	Chin-ups (11)	Dips (31)
Triceps press down (110x13)	Shrugs, dumbbell (87/arm x12)	Biceps curls (90x12 - bar)
Pull-ups / pull-downs* (155x12)	Calf raises (205x9)	Overhead cable triceps extension (60x10)
Chest cable fly (190x8)	Squats (175x8)	Squats (175x7)
Deadlifts (245x10)	Dumbbell lateral raise (22.5x10)	Shrugs, dumbbell (80/arm x12)
Rows (160x12)	Overhead cable triceps extension (60x12)	Curls (90x12)
Metabolic finisher (bike @ 25x, 30s)	Overhead press, barbell (85x12)	Bench or chest press (155x6, 135x6)
+ Add another card	Leg extension (350x11)	Pull-ups / pull-downs* (142.5x13)
	Metabolic finisher (bike @ 25x, 25s)	Leg extension (340x12)
	+ Add another card	Overhead press, barbell (70x14)
		Shrugs, dumbbell (80/arm x10)
		Dips (30)
		Dips (28)
		Leg extension (325x15)
		Pull-ups / pull-downs* (140x11)
		+ Add another card

For unfamiliar readers, Trello is a free tool that digitizes the well-known workflow management style known as Kanban. If you've ever made a series of to-do lists, where a given to-do's status moves from the left to the right as it nears completion, you are already familiar with Kanban.

Sign up for Trello and make a board "Fitness" with lists A-Day, B-Day, and Gains. You can also make a copy of **this template**.

MYFITNESSPAL / LOSEIT!

As a long-time user of both, I don't have a strong recommendation over either option.

These apps make it easy to monitor what you're eating and add a lot of color to the "why" you might be asking yourself when you step on a scale and don't weigh what you *think you ought to*. Calorie tracker apps essentially prevent denial, and force you to be honest with yourself about what goes into your body.

If you fast intermittently, stop snacking, and have mostly predictable, boring meals, it will be painless to stay in sync with your calorie tracker of choice.

For those who don't travel much and have a consistent routine at home, you can safely stop using these apps after 60-90 days of diligence and reflection. If you're like me and you travel frequently, I strongly recommend the daily ounce of pain—5-10 mins tops—to log all of your meals. And since you're fasting, you'll only have 1-2 meals to log anyway.

Sometimes you'll forget to log a meal immediately after it happens, or you won't be able to find the exact ingredient in your food tracker's library. Don't sweat it. What I like to do is pick something that's definitely *more* caloric, fatty, or carb-filled, then vow to eat cleaner next time.

The other thing we'll use is a calorie tracker for progress pics.

Export	Progress	+

⌇	Weight	☑	2 Months

196.6 lbs	**176.8 lbs**	**⬇ 19.8 lbs**
START	CURRENT	CHANGE (-10.1%)

195

190

185

180

176.8

12/23   12/30   1/6   1/13   1/20   1/27   2/3   2/10   2/17

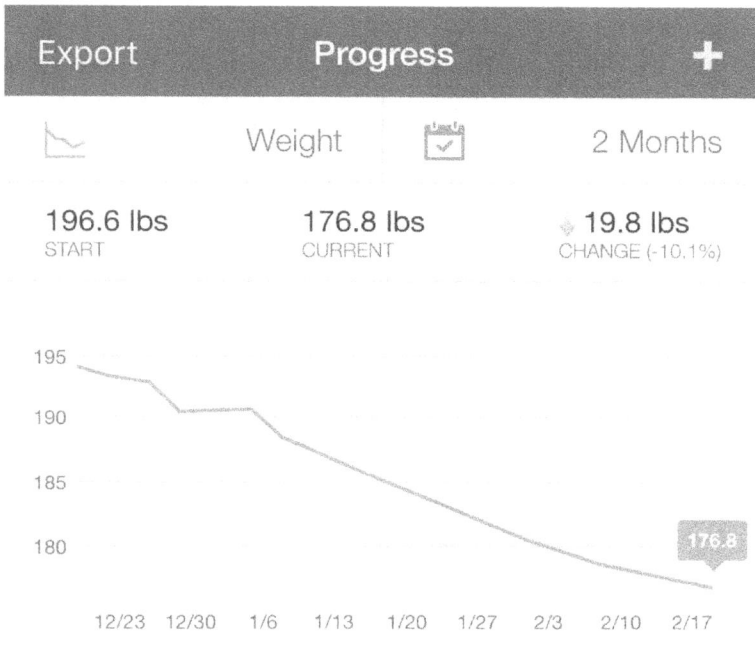

Whenever you hit "log," you get the option to choose foods or workouts or weight or pics. Once a week, usually on Sundays, I try to weigh-in at a gym and attach my updated mass in pounds plus a candid selfie directly into MyFitnessPal. Your first couple of progress pics will be the most dramatic, but you should keep taking them anyway because body composition changes are more subtle over time. Without these pictures, all the metrics in the world might not motivate you to continue.

GOOGLE SHEETS

We already explained why weight is a singular variable in the path to becoming your best self. To temper our motivation, we'll also track our body composition and, thus, discover potential fat loss or less-visible muscle gain in the process.

At least 2 times per month (I do it once /week alongside my weigh-in), log the circumference of your arms, legs, neck, belly, and chest. These metrics go into the same worksheet you copied earlier, and produce a simple graph over time.

	A	B	C	D	E	F	G
	date	R arm	L arm	R leg	L leg	neck	bellybutton
	Jan 6	13.188	13.125	21.750	21.688	14.250	33.813
	Jan 13	13.000	13.500	21.000	21.500	14.250	33.688
	Jan 20	13.000	13.055	20.688	21.013	14.500	33.250
	Jan 27	12.938	13.313	19.000	20.500	14.500	32.125

I've hard-coded the "estimated" weight loss per week to just 2 pounds. This is a generic doctor-approved recommendation and also very achievable. Pending how much weight you have to lose, you'll likely see a 3+ pound mass reduction in as little as 7 days by following this program, but I do not recommend updating the "estimated" weekly weight loss.

Enjoy the ride "below the wave" when it happens, but understand your body shreds "edge node fats" with a lot less effort than the type of fat you really want to get rid of: that tire around your belly button. While everyone's body is unique, for me, those "edge node fats" include my upper legs, neck, and cheeks. That fat falls off, whereas the abdomen region, not so much.

We'll discuss exactly how to measure your body composition in a later chapter to reduce false positives and false negatives caused by poor timing or inflammation.

IS THIS REALLY NECESSARY?

Spartans long before us got ripped without any software or even awareness of the ketogenic diet. They also didn't have cars and air conditioning to keep them comfortable in between training sessions.

Even most modern approaches to fitness don't ask for this degree of digital tracking, but that's why most approaches to fitness aren't a sustainable option for hackers like you. This is not a "first-time fitness plan," it's a "I've tried the normal stuff, what the hell" call to arms.

Tracking calories, how much you can bench press, and whether or not you snacked last night might sound silly at first. That's OK, feel silly. If you are unwilling to do this for just 90 days, you will *look* silly forever.

HARDWARE

With our tech stack out of the way, it's time to make a couple more commitments to yourself.

1. you need access to a GYM
2. see #1

YouTube is littered with 1,000's of at-home workouts you can do with little to no equipment. These are great if your goal is simply endurance and cardio, but weight loss and muscle gain are a lot easier if you eat right and lift weights.

When author and filmmaker Mike Cernovich interviewed Dr. Brett Osborn, a board-certified neurosurgeon, for his book *Gorilla Mindset*, Brett's clinical opinion on this was quite clear:

> Mike: If I only have time to do cardio or lift, what should I do?
> Dr. Osborn: Without question lift weights. I would rather see a healthy person do 50 squats a day than walk a mile… Lifting weights improves your muscular structure, boosts your immune system, and does not provide excess stress hormones like cortisol (some running and other long-duration cardio can do).

Dr. Osborn outlines more of these convictions in his book *Get Serious*.[12]

If you're already a member of a gym, great. But if you aren't, or you are but are unhappy, consider this the final step in your Fitness for Hackers onboarding.

Here are your fitness center options.

Tier 1 ($125+ /month)
Typically the largest gyms in your area and where "rich" people go to work out. Well-Kept locker rooms, showers, free classes (boxing / cycling / etc.) included in the membership. Not uncommon for these gyms to have spas, pools, and a sauna or steam room in the locker rooms.

Tier 2 ($40 - $100 /month)
Co-Ed locker area, more advanced machines, and duplication (i.e. multiple bench presses for busy hours). Personal trainers on-site but not required. Possibly pushy sales and membership process.

Tier 3 ($9 - $25 /month)
No-Frills, weights and machines only. Sometimes accessible 24/7.

At every gym, there are serious people and tire-kickers. Some chains have brands that attract certain characters, thus, Gold's Gym might have more "meat heads" than say, Lifetime or Anytime Fitness. We'll talk about handling this later so you can stay focused on #1, you.

I personally pay top dollar for a Tier 1 gym. However, during my fitness "kick" periods, I had success at Tier 2 and Tier 3 gyms as well. Even apartment gyms are theoretically good enough to get the job done, although I don't recommend it if you can afford a membership elsewhere. Think about it: apartment gyms are almost always empty. They're so convenient you can always go later (i.e. never).

If you're struggling to justify joining a gym, put down this book and enjoy a piece of cake instead.

IN DEFENSE OF EXPENSIVE GYMS

The hackers I know are successful.

They can buy the latest MacBook, travel internationally, support their family, and give back to their communities. If this sounds like you, perhaps you need a "push" to decide if it's responsible to pay more for a gym when a cheap one will suffice.

Here's why I personally prefer "fancy" gyms:

- logistics → going to the gym is NEVER convenient, but you can reduce back/forth to your home or car or office by picking a gym with decent showers
- people → when I lived in Harlem I joined a $9 /month gym and was reminded that you "get what you pay for." a few usual suspects were notorious for leaving sweaty rags on the gear to claim a machine as their territory. I often had to wait a few minutes between each lift simply to avoid conflict.
- equipment → I joined a "meat head" type gym in Busan, South Korea, during my 2-week stay on Haeundae Beach. The bench press, squat rack, and other quintessential machines were old and rusty, and I actually sliced open my left ankle (yes blood) while moving around the floor. Bad or old equipment is sharp, and you're more likely to collide with something that isn't padded or safe.
- enthusiasm → if your body is a temple, the gym is a body's temple. Paying more for a pleasant atmosphere will encourage you to still make it, even on your "off" days.

The choice is yours, but it's smart to consider how much money you spend on superfluous crap before scoffing at a monthly membership rate. If I personally ate 1 fewer steak dinner per month, that's a membership at most gyms.

SCIENCE AND GYMS

Welcome to the 3rd argument that urges you to invest in yourself with a nice gym membership. German psychologist Kurt Lewin backs me up with a simple formula known as Lewin's Equation.[13]

$$B = f(P, E)$$

This says *Behavior* is a function of *Person* and their *Environment*. Kids who hang out with drug dealers become drug dealers. Young professionals who host meetings at happy hours, drink. People who go to brunch, wear Sperry boat shoes.

Hackers who work out alongside other people who are serious about their health are healthier. And this principle applies to the good stuff (workouts) as well as the bad (free donuts). You will behave according to your environment.

PART I SUMMARY

I spent 3 chapters telling you my story and setting us up for success over the next 90 days.

Before moving on to Part II:

- set a goal, then reduce the scope to make it achievable within 3 months
- download and familiarize yourself with the tools I introduced (Trello, calorie counter, Zero, strength worksheet)
- if you don't have a gym membership, get one or stop reading this book

PART I NOTES

1. *"I have not failed. I've just found 10,000 ways that won't work."*
    — Thomas Edison
2. Satire of the Rifleman's Creed, created by Major General William H. Rupertus during WWII. Many popular open
    source libraries also reference it.
3. Donald Watson and veganism, https://www.dictionary.com/e/veganism/
4. https://www.lindtusa.com/wcsstore/LindtCatalogAssetStore/Attachment/products/nutritional/nutritional-information-SKU-438281.pdf
5. https://www.lindtusa.com/wcsstore/LindtCatalogAssetStore/Attachment/products/nutritional/nutritional-information-SKU-392977.pdf
6. https://www.popsugar.com/fitness/How-Much-Sugar-Can-You-Have-Keto-Diet-45266172
7. Wonder Bread nutrition, https://www.fooducate.com/app#!page=product&id=556190A2-32C7-11E3-A74D-1E047F0525AB
8. https://www.verywellfit.com/walking-calories-burned-by-miles-3887154
9. this rule is inspired by Winston Churchill: https://www.independent.co.uk/news/uk/home-news/my-dear-you-are-ugly-but-tomorrow-i-shall-be-sober-and-you-will-still-be-ugly-winston-churchill-tops-8878622.html
10. https://www.amazon.com/48-Laws-Power-Robert-Greene/dp/0140280197/

11. Gollwitzer, P. M. (1999). Implementation intentions: Strong effects of simple plans. American Psychologist, 54, 493-503

12. *Get Serious* by Dr Brett Osborn https://www.amazon.com/dp/B00J4BK96Q/

13. Lewin's Equation, https://u.osu.edu/studentemployment/2015/01/28/bfpe/, published 1936 by Kurt Lewin

PART II

ACTIVATION

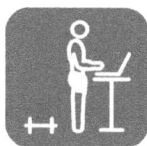

CHAPTER 4

PERFORMANCE BENCHMARKS

"I already know what giving up feels like. I want to see what happens if I don't."
— Neila Rey

Whenever a programming language gets a version bump, developers pounce on the opportunity to run performance benchmarks.

Ana Gómez, a mathematician and Ruby core contributor, introduced her 2 new Array methods `.union()` and `.difference()` to Ruby 2.6 by announcing[1] them on her blog:

> [1, 3, 5, 7, 9].**union**([2, 3, 4, 5, 6]) #=> *[1, 3, 5, 7, 9, 2, 4, 6]*
> [1, 1, 3, 3, 5, 7, 9].**difference**([3, 4, 7]) #=> *[1, 1, 5, 9]*
>
> Array#union is also equivalent to combine Array#concat and Array#uniq (with the difference that concat modifies the array), but more readable. But what is really important about those new methods, are the gains in efficiency when having more than two arrays.

We need some Benchmarks now. (*emphasis mine*)

Using Array.new(num_elements){Random.rand(20_100_000)} to create four arrays with 20,000,000, 30,000,000, 8,000,000 and 25,000,000 elements, those are the times for the different options:

- (array1 | array2 | array3 | array4) ~ 20.043 seconds
- array1.union(array2, array3, array4) ~ 13.390 seconds
- array1.concat(array2, array3, array4).uniq ~ 20.633 seconds

So please, stop using concat + uniq

If we nerd out on methods that save a few seconds at runtime, doesn't it make sense to do the same for our body? Especially when we can add *years*—not seconds—to our lifespan?

UNKNOWN UNKNOWNS

By now, you've downloaded a calorie tracker app and added your last meal. It's OK if doing that feels depressing… your next meal log won't. You should have also measured your body and recorded those values in the metrics worksheet provided in Chapter 3.

I personally have an **OrbiTape**, which makes it easy to measure yourself without a friend or partner's assistance. While traveling, I use a smaller, also retractable version, but it doesn't "catch" the other end. To ensure accuracy—measuring each of my muscles and ligaments from the same spot—my wife assists in this weekly check-in.

But while your weight, caloric intake, and muscle size are enough to understand *aesthetic* changes and anecdotal observations of your energy and physical comfort, you will inevitably hit a plateau on your journey. Tracking at least 1 of the following "invisible" metrics will help you conquer those periods.

Invisible fitness metrics include:

- BMI (Body Mass Index, relationship of fat to height and weight)
- Body Composition (overall fitness level)
- BMR (Basal Metabolic Rate, how many calories you burn in a resting state)
- Ketones (ketone bodies, created when your body burns fat instead of muscle, accelerated by low-carb diets)
- Body Fat % (what portion of your mass is fat, includes "essential" and "storage")
- FMS[2] (Functional Movement Screen, degree of mobility across 7 disciplines and scored 0-3 each)

Understanding where you stand in all of these dimensions is overkill if this is your first serious attempt at personal fitness. Further, gathering these results can be expensive or inconvenient based on your proximity to capable facilities.

For this reason, exploring invisible metrics is an optional part of the Fitness for Hackers program. I do recommend, however, being evaluated for at least 1 or 2 of these metrics. At a minimum, get a DXA scan to measure your body composition.

DXA SCAN

In September 2015, I became fed up with being "only a marketer" in New York City, so I listed my studio apartment on Airbnb and bought a 1-way ticket to Chiang Mai, Thailand. I planned to attempt to learn how to code, then maybe fail (not smart enough?) and move to Dallas, Texas, where my girlfriend was working at this time.

Fast forward a few months, I parlayed my new tech skills into an operational role at a venture capital fund. I flew halfway around the world again and moved into a brand new San Francisco high rise.

This whirlwind of lifestyle changes led me to experience one of those fitness "kicks" we discussed earlier: a temporal, unsustainable burst of motivation to improve my body.

For a few months, I followed an increasingly popular home workout plan I found online, called Metaconda.[3] Here's how it works:

1. dumbbell swing
2. blast-off Pushup
3. bodyweight squat
4. dumbbell piston push-pull
5. mountain climber
6. hollow-body hold

You do 6 "laps" of the full circuit, spending 30 seconds on each round and doing as many repetitions as you can. The *rub* is that between each round, you rest for 30 seconds, then 25 seconds, then 20… until you want to throw up.

The whole workout takes about 18 minutes, but it was so hard that after a few months, I lost my fire (see: fitness kick). At this point, I clocked another fail in Ryan's fitness diary but was proud enough of my results that I wanted to know what impact it made on my body. All I knew from my own [single variable] measurements was 1 thing: I had lost 10lbs.

That's when I heard about the DXA scan. This technology is an x-ray style scan of your body that measures bone, muscle, and fat density on a per square inch level of granularity.

A quick search introduced me to BodySpec, a mobile scanning company in Los Angeles and San Francisco. I booked an appointment online for $45 and got it done a few days later in their "van" location (seriously). DXA scans take about 10 minutes.

For the enlightened reader, here are a couple notes from that experience. To download my entire original BodySpec report, **go here**.

BODY·SPEC

www.body-spec.com

2148 Federal Ave Suite C
Los Angeles, CA 90025
Phone: (310) 601-8184

Client	Sex	Facility	Birth Date	Height	Weight	Measured
Kulp, Ryan	Male	(not specified)	03/20/1990	71.0 in.	204.0 lbs.	05/10/2016

SUMMARY RESULTS

This table provides an overview of your total body composition, broken down into total body fat %, total mass, fat tissue, lean tissue, and bone mineral content. These metrics establish your baseline from which future BodySpec scans will be compared.

Measured Date	Total Body Fat %	Total Mass (lbs)	Fat Tissue (lbs)	Lean Tissue (lbs)	Bone Mineral Content (BMC)
05/10/2016	21.2%	193.0	40.8	144.3	7.8

Although I was working my butt off in the apartment gym, even supplementing Metaconda workouts with free weights (on good days), my Total Body Fat % was over 20%.

At 193 pounds and 5 feet 11 inches tall, I was nowhere *close* to seeing abs, and this was discouraging. The idea of 30-50 more Metaconda workouts and 6 more months of restricting my eating (no eating at all?) just to lose another 10 pounds felt like a dead-end.

So I responded the only way I knew how when fitness kicks didn't yield the results I wanted: I gave up.

REGIONAL ASSESSMENT

The table below divides your body into 5 key regions and provides the composition breakdown for each. BodySpec automatically tracks these regions over time to chart regional progress and the impact of your training and nutrition programming.

Region	Total Region Fat %	Total Mass (lbs)	Fat Tissue (lbs)	Lean Tissue (lbs)	Bone Mineral Content (BMC)
Arms	17.6%	26.3	4.6	20.5	1.2
Legs	21.4%	72.1	15.4	53.6	3.1
Trunk	22.5%	82.3	18.5	61.6	2.2
Android	22.3%	11.6	2.6	8.9	0.1
Gynoid	25.2%	29.7	7.3	21.7	0.7
Total	21.2%	193.0	40.8	144.3	7.8

In case you think I'm bitter, I'm not. This story is instead a friendly warning. In my case, a DXA scan ironically *hurt* my motivation to continue exploring my fitness potential.

I was self-righteous about the mental toughness I exhibited in my apartment's basement gym, and I allowed a machine to let me think *"a great body just isn't something I'm capable of having."*

The implications here are unnerving, as my typical personality is marked by self-prophecy and making your own luck. But in the fitness realm, I relegated my mindset to a fixed, scarcity-based, victim mentality.

Through this process, I learned humans are simultaneously capable of being victims or victors, it just depends on the context. You might be a sought after CTO yet simultaneously afraid of talking to women, for example. You could have an excellent work ethic in your knowledge work, but a terrible work ethic in your dieting or gym discipline. Perhaps, one day, "excellence" will be transferable, but until then, we have to re-develop the strengths that come naturally to us in each modality it is required.

DXA SCAN PRO TIP

If you're a data nerd like me and agree that DXA scans pack a lot of insights, I encourage you to schedule a DXA scan this week and then do a follow-up in 3 months. Don't wait for results first. See where you are now so you can understand your progress.

Most providers, including BodySpec, combine your previous results with new exams, so there's a compounding interest effect to going more than once. BodySpec even offers a small discount to book 2 exams upfront for exactly this purpose.

DXA SCAN ALTERNATIVE

Let's return to the topic of expense. While good health is theoretically price-less, we all have very real budgets and incomes that can be dedicated to other good things in our lives besides our bodies.

If you're craving scientific results but aren't willing or able to spend $45+ on a DXA scan, see if you can find an InBody machine instead.

In Hanoi, Vietnam, I was able to get an exam done for just $2 USD, which included a printout of my results.

TRUNG TÂM ECOFIT NGOẠI GIAO ĐOÀN
73 Vạn Bảo, Ngọc Khánh, Ba Đình, Hà Nội
Tel: 043.9562222 / 043.9563333 Hotline: 096.996 5151
Website: www.ecofit.vn Email: ecofitcenter73vanbao@gmail.com

ECOFIT CENTER

[InBody270]

ID	Height	Age	Gender	Date	Time
6 165436528	180. 3cm	8	Male	2019.03.11.	14:32

Body Composition Analysis

Total Body Water — 52. 4 (40. 2~49. 2)
Protein — 14. 3 (10. 8~13. 2)
Mineral — 4. 65 (3. 72~4. 54)
Body Fat Mass — 7. 5 (8. 6~17. 2)
Weight (kg) — 78. 9 (60. 8~82. 2)

InBody Score

91 /100 Points

* Total score that reflects the evaluation of body composition. A muscular person may score over 100 points.

Weight Control

Target Weight 78. 9 kg
Weight Control 0. 0 kg
Fat Control 0. 0 kg
Muscle Control 0. 0 kg

Obesity Evaluation

BMI ☑Normal ☐Under ☐Slightly Over / ☐Over
PBF ☑Normal ☐Slightly Over ☐Over

Muscle Fat Analysis

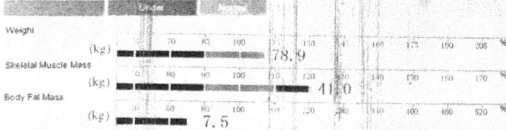

Weight (kg) 78. 9
Skeletal Muscle Mass (kg) 41. 0
Body Fat Mass (kg) 7. 5

Waist-Hip Ratio
0. 82 0. 80 0. 90

Visceral Fat Level
Level 2 Low 10 High

Obesity Analysis

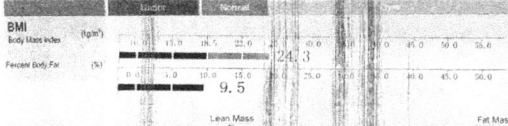

BMI Body Mass Index (kg/m²) 24. 3
Percent Body Fat (%) 9. 5

Research Parameters

Fat Free Mass 71. 4 kg
Basal Metabolic Rate 1912 kcal
Obesity Degree 110 % (90~110)
Recommended calorie intake 2868 kcal

Calorie Expenditure of Exercise

Golf	139	Gateball	150
Walking	158	Yoga	158
Badminton	178	Table Tennis	178
Tennis	237	Bicycling	237
Boxing	237	Basketball	237
Mountain Climbing	257	Jumping Rope	276
Aerobics	276	Jogging	276
Soccer	276	Swimming	276
Japanese Fencing	395	Racketball	395
Squash	395	Taekwondo	395

* Based on your current weight
* Based on 30 minute duration

Segmental Lean Analysis
Lean Mass % Evaluation

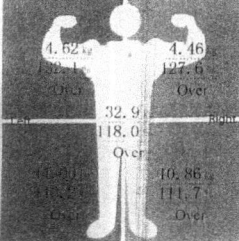

Segmental Fat Analysis
Fat Mass % Evaluation

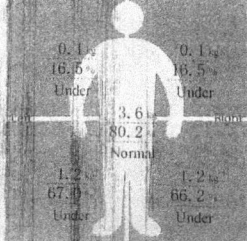

* Segmental fat is estimated.

Results Interpretation QR Code

Scan the QR Code to see results interpretation in more detail.

Impedance

Z (Ω) | RA | LA | TR | RL | LL
20 kHz | 264. 4 | 234. 7 | 20. 4 | 228. 3 | 220. 1
100 kHz | 215. 1 | 208. 2 | 17. 4 | 197. 6 | 189. 3

Body Composition History

Weight (kg) 78. 9
Skeletal Muscle Mass (kg) 41. 0
Percent Body Fat (%) 9. 5

▼ Recent □ Total

For context, this scan was done after just 12 weeks of my Fitness for Hackers regimen and during the morning following a Japanese steak buffet dinner.

My key takeaways from the InBody exam:

- at just 9.5% body fat, I'm in the zone for 6-pack abs
- since I don't yet *have* well-defined abs, I should focus more on core workouts than losing more weight
- my BMR (basal metabolic rate) is 1,900 calories, which explains my safe and sustainable 1-2 pounds per week weight loss at a caloric restriction of 1,650 calories per day

Download a copy of my InBody results **here**.

FINDING INSIGHTS IN YOUR BLOOD KETOSIS

Of all the invisible metrics available, body fat % and ketones are the only 2 I personally measure on a regular basis.

If you're experimenting with a low-carb diet like me, it's helpful and motivating (or soul-crushing) to know whether you're actually *pulling it off*.

For example, I mentioned earlier that sauces at restaurants often have sugar in them. Well, they also have carbs. So while you might not physically eat a piece of bread in your new diet, and may become highly skilled in saying "no rice please" at your next fajita night out, carbs are *everywhere*.

To determine whether you're actually eating < 30 grams (my suggestion) or < 50 net grams of carbohydrates per day, pick up a box of **Ketostix**[4] (< $15). You pee on them, and they change color based on how many ketone bodies are detected in your body. To support my friend's startup that competes with Ketostix, try **Perfect Keto Strips**[5] instead.

Since 25+ strips come in a box, you only need to do this a few times to understand and reveal your true eating habits. After measuring myself every day for a few weeks straight, I stopped taking them. Again, boring and replicable meals help reduce mental clutter, and you do not need to make ketone body testing a regular part of your schedule.

REFACTORING YOUR GOALS

A better understanding of invisible health metrics might compel you to modify the goal you set in Chapter 3. For example, if your goal was to lose 15lbs, you might now prefer to extend that goal with "reach < 15% body fat."

Refactoring your initial, single-dimensional goal could result in the following:

1. lose weight
2. lose *more* weight to hit sub-15% body fat (stretch goal)

But an even better approach looks like this:

1. lose weight see my own abs
2. acknowledge sub-10% body fat is a prerequisite[6] for abs visibility
3. ⇒ calculate how much weight I should lose to see my abs AND achieve X% body fat

Here's a guide from the American Council on Exercise (ACE) on general ranges of body fat % that are reasonable for men and women, grouped by your intended body type:

Description	Women	Men
Essential fat	10–13%	3–5%
Athletes	14–20%	6–13%
Fitness	21–24%	14–17%
Average	25–31%	18–24%
Obese	32%+	25%+

Essential fat is a metric that, should you dip below, could result in your exit from the gene pool. In other words, a physically fit person in the Fitness cohort really only has around 10% "storage" body fat.

The hard truth from my San Francisco story is that while I was dieting OK and working out hard, my results (21.2% body fat) were nothing more than *average*.

Thoughtfully considering what you actually want vs. what sounds good on paper (HIT, circuit training, etc.) will help you apply this book's fitness plan to be more prescriptive to your goals. And to know whether you've achieved those goals, set benchmarks.

DAY 1 - FITNESS FOR HACKERS

It's time to hit the gym.

Unlike personal trainers who focus on making you lose your breath to satisfy their sense of self-worth, I'm going to walk you through how to take it easy on Day 1 in the gym.

Here's all we need to understand before our 2nd, more rigorous workout:

1. How to perceive ourselves and others in the weight room / locker room
2. What the hell each machine does
3. How much weight we should be lifting

GYM ANXIETY

Remember your first hackathon when you felt like an imposter? Maybe your first internship or standup?

When you walk into the gym for the first time or even the fiftieth time, it's normal to feel like everyone is staring and judging you. Maybe your shoes look a little too "new" or your gym bag is too fancy, or your workout shirt is too bright to have possibly been washed before.

Here's the thing: all those judgments I just described are coming from *you*. The fact is, nobody actually cares. Most people go to the gym to "do their time" and then purge the entire memory, from who they saw to even what they *did*, the moment they walk out of the door.

Sure, there might be a couple snickering losers who "live" in the gym because they don't have marketable skills or a personality IRL, but they're just projecting insecurities. If you experience someone like this, understand the only thing they know for sure is you have more important things to do outside the gym than they do.

Dr. Rick Kattouf, a fitness and nutrition expert, says this about so-called "*Gymphobia*:"[7]

> "*Any apprehension, intimidation and insecurity an individual may feel when they walk in is self-imposed," he notes. "No one else cares. Seriously, they don't. When a weight-room veteran sees a newbie come in, we say, 'Good for them, glad to see them lifting weights.'*"

With this out of the way, let's lift weights.

MACHINES ARE JUST TOOLS

In tech, we have dozens, 100s, maybe 1000s of tools that can be combined in a million ways to get the job done.

To a layman, these tools look identical… MySQL, PostgreSQL. But depending on our needs, one could be a 10x better implementation decision. The same goes at the gym.

Everything you see on the gym floor, from machines to free weights, creates either *isolated* or *compound* stress for your body.

Two examples:

- dumbbell, the 10 inch wide hand-held free weights with octagonal end-caps → isolated, for Biceps
- kettlebell, the sphere free weights with an upside-down U shaped handle → compound, for Core / Shoulders

An isolated lift *isolates* resistance to a single muscle. A compound lift simply combines 2 or more isolated lifts into a single movement. Often the affected muscles are in the same "muscle group," or for our purposes, body zone.

Isolation tools (free weights) can also be used for compound exercises, e.g. you can curl a dumbbell with your right hand, starting at your waist (knuckles touching your right thigh) and then (when the weight is close to your chest) "press" the weight straight up toward the ceiling.

This movement puts stress on both your biceps (part 1, the curl) as well as your shoulders or deltoids.

In our Hackers fitness plan, we'll focus primarily on isolated lifts for two reasons:

1. it's easier to remember your sequences, thus more sustainable
2. every muscle in every body grows at a different pace

Regarding #2, suppose you enjoy a compound lift entailing bicep curls to your chest, followed immediately by a military press (pushing the weights to the ceiling). It's likely that while your biceps may only be able to handle, say, 30 pounds, your shoulders could be much stronger and able to handle 40 or 50 pounds of resistance.

As you can see, being "too efficient" in your workout actually limits the potential of your muscles by making each one dependent on the strength of another. Isolated workouts let us avoid this by affording each muscle its own Product Strength Roadmap.

With this in mind, here are the tools we need to be comfortable using at the gym:

- dumbbells → versatile, hand-held, come in all sizes from 2 pounds to 100+ pounds /each
    o can be used for biceps, triceps, obliques, forearms, deltoids, lats, and chest
- barbells → the wide, 4 to 5 feet long (1-2 meters) metal bars without weight on them
    o great for shoulders, chest, squats, deadlifts
    o also an alternative to dumbbell for biceps and triceps if you prefer to synchronize your left / right arm curls
- pulley machine → complicated looking rack with pulleys, sometimes a chin-up bar, and lots of straps hanging out
    o my preferred tool for triceps (via "press downs" which we'll cover) and pull-ups / chin-ups
- rowing machine → the long bench with interchangeable handlebars and foot pads
    o as the name implies, you "row" weight by pulling toward yourself; works middle and lower back
- dip machine → sometimes a raised pair of "arm pads" five feet off the ground, sometimes a sit-down device
    o also triceps and deltoids, this is one of my favorite singular exercises to monitor progress over time

There are dozens of other tools in the gym; we don't need any of them right now.

Legendary football player Herschel Walker claims[8] he *never* lifted weights, opting instead for 3,500 pushups and sit-ups every day. During an interview with NFL in 2015, he says this:

> *"I grew up overweight… I used to have a speech impediment. I was picked on. And I realized that if you dedicate yourself to anything, you can do it. "Still doing no weights. Everything has been body exercises. Almost like a gymnast. I can do the rings. I can do that pommel horse. And people are shocked that I can do it. "Almost everybody wants to look like a bodybuilder and do 500 pounds on the bench. That sounds good, but all of sudden you've got back problems and all these other problems."*

So no, we don't need more tools… yet. In Part III of this book, we'll explore advanced techniques you can add to your routine, but think of those as addendums. What's next in Chapter 5 is more than enough for your 90-day experiment, and is essentially a replica of the plan that led me to 24+ pounds weight loss (196 to 172) in just 11 weeks.

BUT WHAT ABOUT CARDIO?

I mentioned previously that we're not going to worry about cardio. Unless you're one of the few blessed creatures who enjoy running, it actually really sucks and is more likely to lead to you quitting your plan altogether.

In 2019 we don't have to run away from predators (unless you're in The Tenderloin), and we have bikes, cars, electric scooters, and Craigslist to get us around.

Again, in Part III, I'll introduce optional cardio enhancements you can bolt on to your workout routine, but first, let's get you eating right and in the gym twice per week.

Yes, just twice, and for no more than 30 minutes each time.

HOW TO SET YOUR FITNESS BENCHMARKS

On your first visit to the gym, we simply want to log our approximate "max" lift values in the Trello you set up earlier. As a reminder, this should have 3 lists on a "Fitness" board that looks like this:

A-Day	B-Day	Gains

Inside of our A-Day and B-Day lists, we're going to add 7-10 lifts. You can consider the sum of those lifts a "sequence." the Fitness for Hackers sequence is what's commonly called an A/B schedule, and later we'll add an optional C-Day for the insane readers among you.

A simple example is to work out your arms in A-Day and legs in B-Day. But we can get a little "closer to the metal" than that and work out different parts of our arms, chest, back, and shoulders on both days. I shared the differences between isolated and compound lifts is for this reason: we want to isolate the muscles used during one sequence, so they have ample time to recover during the other sequence.

Here's the overview:

- our A-Day will focus on biceps, triceps, chest, and butt.
- our B-Day will focus on lats, thighs, calves, shoulders, and back.

In both sequences, there will be overlap, but soreness will be kept to a minimum. Now let's set up your A-Day together.

Walk over to the free weight rack or a "bicep / curling" sit-down machine. Pick up a single 20-pound dumbbell and face the mirror. If you work in kilograms, 7.5kg (16.53 pounds) is more likely in stock.

Standing with your back straight, but without locking your knees, hold the barbell beside your body and squeeze the handle tight. Your arm should be straight by your sides. Finally, "curl" the weight toward your chest over a 4-6 second period.

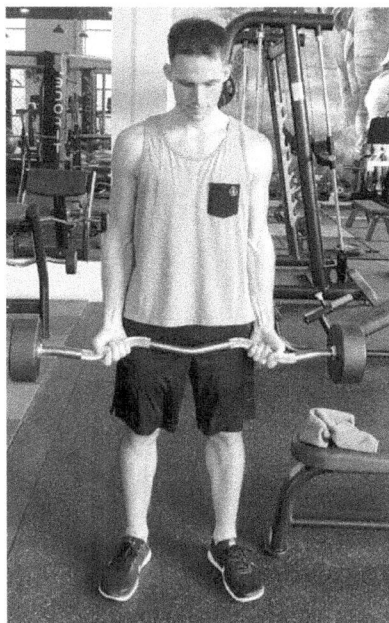

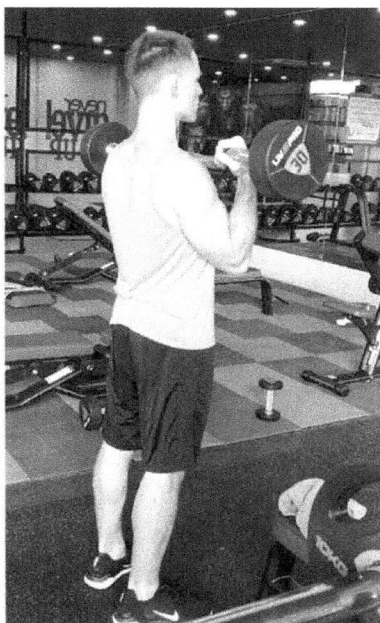

Note the resistance of the weight you chose. Do you think you could do 5 more of those? How about 25 more? Sensing this is critical, and you're about to learn why.

LIFT TO FAILURE MATH

Here's a quick way to calculate how much weight you should be lifting. With a given mass, if you think you could easily do 10 more repetitions of the lift, increase the resistance (weight) until you think you can only do 6-10 sequential repetitions. This means you're saying: on repetition N, I would give up and need to physically drop the weight.

For me, this meant picking up a 25-pound dumbbell (the small hand-held weight), then increasing to 50lbs, then back to 40lbs, for one arm. Within a few weeks I was comfortable lifting 45 to 50 pounds per arm simultaneously, but to protect my form I switched from per-hand dumbbells to a 3-foot wide barbell (depicted here), with which I now curl 90 pounds total, 14 reps straight.

Important gotcha: narrow barbells (3 feet) usually weigh 25 pounds standalone, and wide barbells (5 feet, used for bench press / squats / deadlifts) usually weight 45 pounds standalone. So, curling 45 pounds per arm → 90 pounds total → is achieved by adding just 65 pounds in "plates," or 32.5 pounds to each side of the narrow barbell.

After completing this process for the isolated bicep curl, make a Trello card in your tracker like this:

A-Day
Bicep curls (60x8)

Obviously use pounds or kilograms, whatever floats your bloat. The convention is simple:

```
{{ muscle }} {{ lift }} ({{ weight }} x {{ repetitions }})
```

If you prefer a bit more granularity, try my method of also appending the specific style of lift, i.e. "bar" vs. "dumbbell:"

```
{{ muscle }} {{ lift }} ({{ weight }} x {{ repetitions }} - bar)
```

Two reasons it's important to know if you used a bar or dumbbell:

1. dumbbell implies *per arm or leg*, so seeing "50" implies your left arm lifts 50 and your right arm lifts 50
2. biceps and triceps, in particular, leave a lot of "room" for bad posture, and you'd be amazed to see the difference between what you *think* you

can curl (usually via dumbbells) vs. what you can actually curl (via barbell)

Point #2 speaks to something any seasoned lifter will call you out on if you let them: *swinging*.

If you use your body weight and existing momentum from a given lift's motion to "propel" the next repetition toward its completion, you're cheating yourself. A slower lift (smooth up and down directions) deters swinging weight around and thinking you are stronger than you really are.

REFACTORING YOUR FIRST LIFT

You've now tracked your optimal bicep curl of, say, 25 pounds per arm and 8 repetitions each. In 2 gym visits from now, you'll do this lift *for real*, and you need to do it 8 times straight as you promised yourself you would.

Before moving on, consider if 25 pounds and 8 repetitions (or whatever values you established) is realistic given the handful of other lifts you'll also need to accomplish in a single workout. If you're not at least 90% confident you can hit all your numbers, reduce your estimated repetition count by 1 or 2.

A-DAY BENCHMARKS CONTINUED

Once you're satisfied with the resistance (weight) and repetitions for your bicep curl lift, it's time to move on to the other lifts in our A-Day sequence.

They are:

- dips
- tricep press downs
- bench press
- pull downs
- chest cable fly

- rows
- deadlifts (optional)

Following are illustrated examples of each lift by this author. For video format, go to fitnessforhackers.com/video-guides.

Remember, Day 1 of Fitness for Hackers is simply a data gathering procedure. You do not want to exhaust yourself, we're just setting benchmarks by which to measure and analyze progress over time.

Next, are lifts I recommend for your initial workout stack. Each is in the following format:

- muscles: parts of your body worked out, where the first listed muscle is the primary beneficiary
- visual: the lift being performed by yours truly
- execution: description of how to perform the lift safely
- notes: considerations for getting started and setting goals

DIPS

muscles:
triceps, shoulders, chest

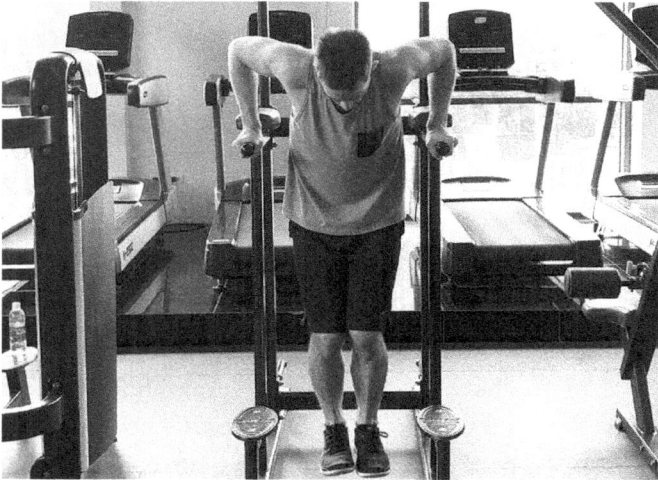

execution:
Stand or sit at the dip machine and grasp the handle bars that protrude out parallel to the floor. Start on the ledge and then let your own body weight "dip" you toward the floor. Your elbows should bend to form a 90-degree angle.

Pending the distance of the dip machine from the ground (many have a riser), you may need to curl your legs up at your knees to prevent your feet from touching the ground.

Some people suggest you stop your descent once your arms are at a 90-degree angle, but as you can see, I prefer to over-extend. This makes it harder to lift myself back up, but also makes your body better than all your peers.

notes:
Try 5 or 10 dips in a row and evaluate how many you think you could do without stopping. I'm currently doing over 40 dips in one set, then I rest a few seconds before my next lift.

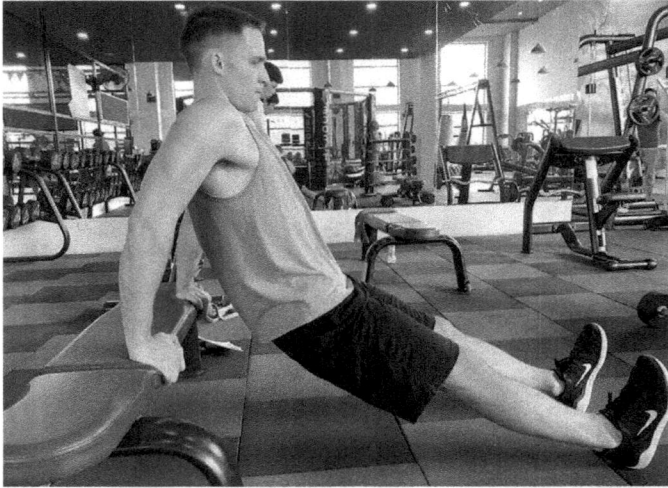

If your gym doesn't have a dip machine, use a raised platform instead. This is also a great alternative for those having trouble lifting their full body weight. If you want the same experience as a dip machine but don't have access to one, multiply your max count by 1.5, and you'll get the same workout.

Since I travel full-time, every week or two means a new country and a new gym membership. Even at respected chains like Anytime Fitness, I had to do 80 dip repetitions in Taipei, Taiwan, because they did not have a dip machine. No biggie.

TRICEP PRESS DOWNS

muscles:
triceps

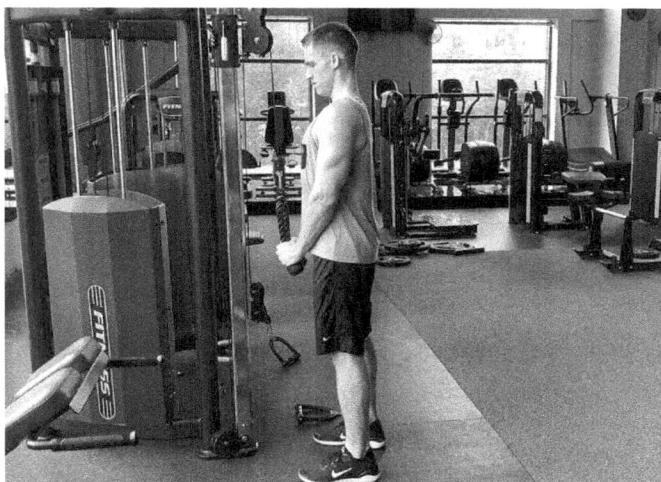

execution:

Attach either a triangular metal handle or black rope style handle to the carabiner shackle attached to the pulley on either side of this machine. Adjust the pulley hardware (usually a pull-out knob, sometimes requires screwing to the left) so the pulley itself is above your head.

With both of your hands holding the ends of your attachment of choice—I usually use the black rope with balled ends—pull down your chosen weight until your arms are completely straight and your hands

are near your knees. A good starting weight is 30 or 40 pounds. I'm currently doing 11 reps straight of 120 pounds total.

notes:

Some pulley machines specify near the weight pins whether the chosen mass amount is per arm or total. If you travel and switch gyms often like I do, and your tricep pull down lift starts to feel too easy, make sure you're not doing half the amount you prescribed in a previous workout session.

BENCH PRESS

muscles:
pectoralis (chest), triceps

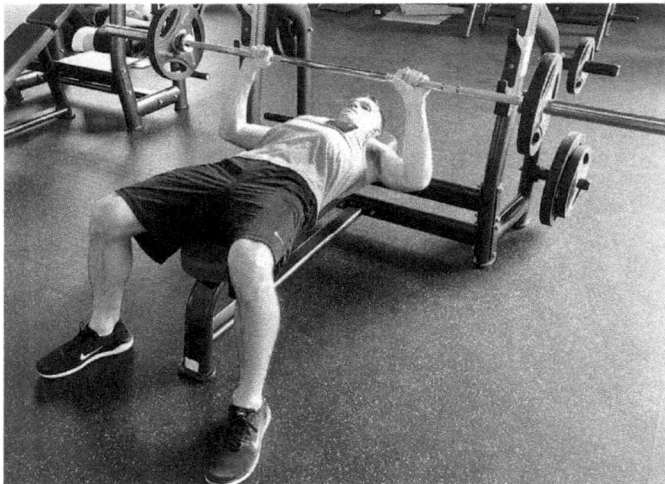

In this illustration, I'm in the middle of a press, but if you watch the videos on fitnessforhackers.com you'll see the bar touches my chest.

execution:
There are 3 ways to angle a chest press: regular, decline, and incline. We'll stick with the flat bench (regular) in our plan, but you're welcome to modify your workout to include incline/decline. These extensions will isolate your upper chest and lower chest, respectively.

notes:
This lift develops our chest and creates *pecs*—you know, the good kind of man boobs. A great way to know if you're lifting too much weight in a chest press is to pay attention to your lower back: it should stay put on the bench. If you find yourself arching your back upwards to finish a press, reduce your resistance or repetition count.

While a barbell and bench is the most common approach to chest press, our "lift to failure" philosophy means it's safer to use a machine. This is because there is no middle "bar" on assisted chest press devices, and thus you can give up at any moment, and all that will happen is a loud "bang." sitting upright at a machine can also help avoid arching your lower back, encouraging better form.

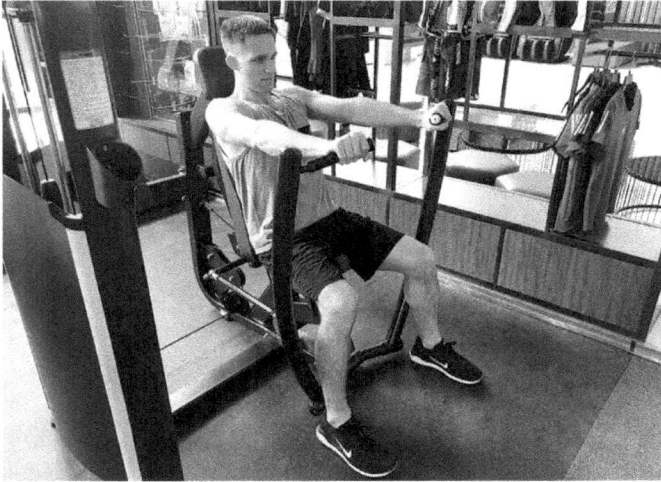

In addition to safety, the bench press machine also helps balance the stress on your muscles.

Lifting near your maximum capacity with a barbell can cause a "wobbly" experience, and you'll end up with one arm or chest muscle stronger and aesthetically bigger than the other. We want symmetry.

PULL DOWNS

muscles:
latissimus dorsi (lats), biceps, forearms

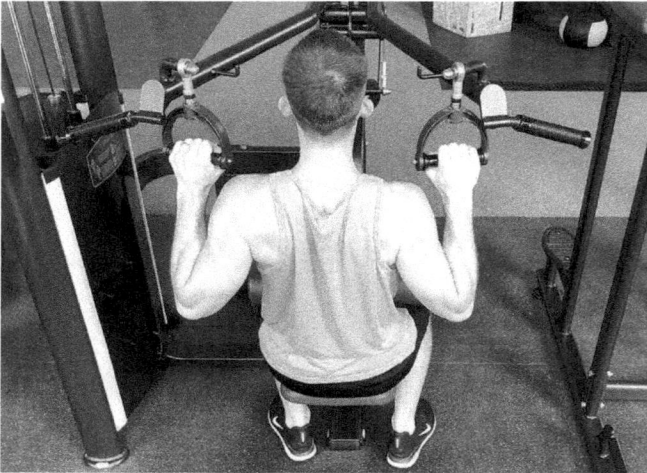

In this illustration, I'm using a machine with free rotating handles, which makes it easier to "place" the stress either in front of or behind your neck. To get a comprehensive workout from this lift, toggle your reps to pull the weight down *in front of* your face (above your chest) as well as behind your head (touching your neck).

execution:
The traditional pull down setup has a weightless bar and adjustable seat. You'll want to set the weight pins on the machine to zero or 10 pounds first, then fix the seat height and knee pads to ensure the bar is in reach before setting your preferred weight.

notes:
This is one of my favorite lifts. Something about pulling vs. pushing feels more natural, and it's easy to adjust the machine to any height or weight you need.

Pull down machines come in a lot of shapes and sizes. Often they're connected to the same Frankenstein machine with which we do tricep pulldowns and rows.

CHEST CABLE FLY

muscles:
pectoralis (pecs)

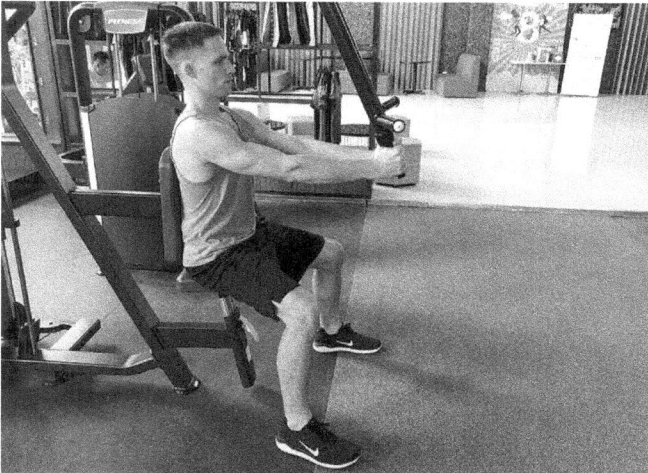

execution:
The traditional bench press has 3 options, including regular, incline, and decline. A fourth approach to this muscle is the chest fly, which works out the sides of our chest and is necessary to have well-rounded man boobs (err pecs). Accomplish this lift by holding your arms closer to your chest, or fully elongated as I do.

In either case, stay consistent between workouts because the amount of weight you'll be able to compress with arms close to your chest is dif-ferent than what you can press with arms fully stretched out.

notes:
Similar to the pull down machine, chest fly machines come in many forms. Some gyms do not have a seated option, so you'll use the same pulley system from our tricep pull down lift, except this time holding one pulley per arm, with the simplest handle you can find.

ROWS

muscles:
latissimus dorsi (back), forearms

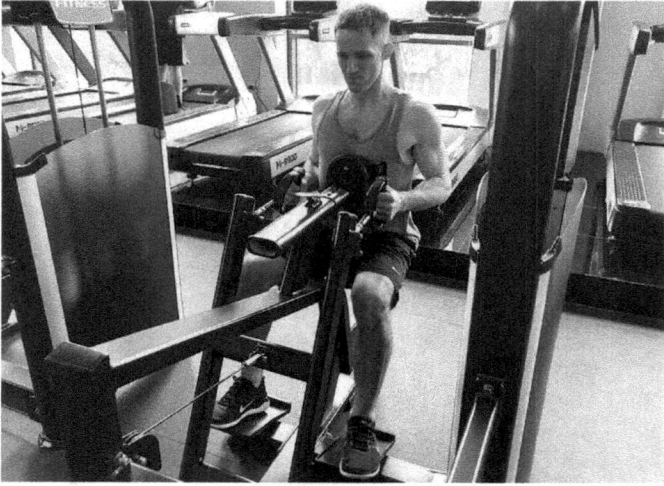

In this illustration, I'm using an assisted row machine that forces my chest and back upright.

execution:
This is as close as we get to a compound lift, by simultaneously working out our back and forearms. With a regular row machine, connected to the multi-purpose pulley and pull down rig, you'll need to watch your form and keep your back straight.

notes:
Some gyms don't have a row machine. I spent 10 days in the Philippines, and my Airbnb gym had a measly 3 machines plus free weights. Refusing to let my muscles deteriorate, I opted into the alternative row that incorporates dumbbells.

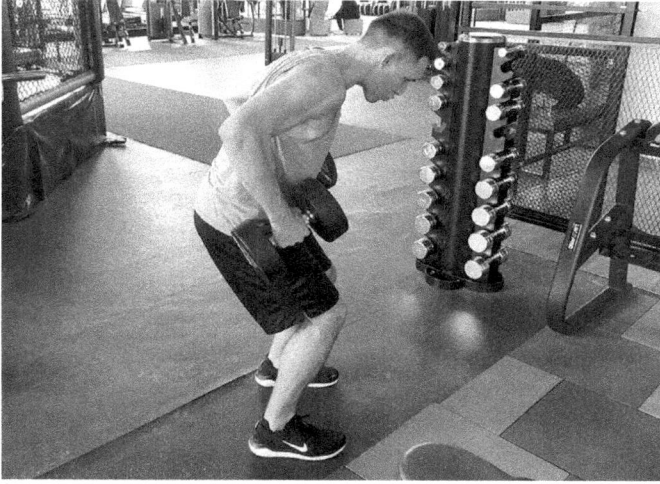

Just like the dip alternative, this is not as ideal as the seated, isolated row that isolates your back. Again we apply the law of contingency and modify our resistance and repetitions accordingly. If your usual set is 140 pounds and 8 repetitions, try a 30-pound dumbbell on each arm and 20 or 30 repetitions in the standing position.

Repeat after me: we never let our gym get in the way of our fitness.[9]

DEADLIFTS (OPTIONAL)

muscles:
lower back, gluteus maximus (butt), hamstrings, finger flexors

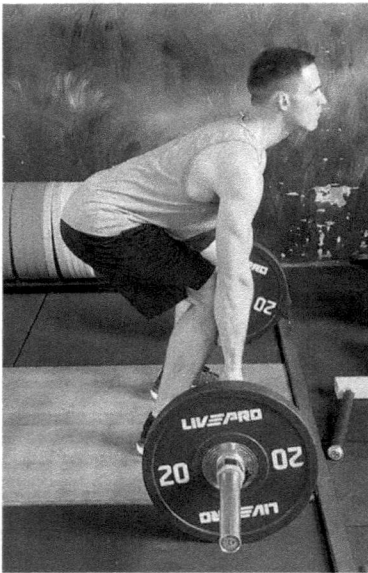

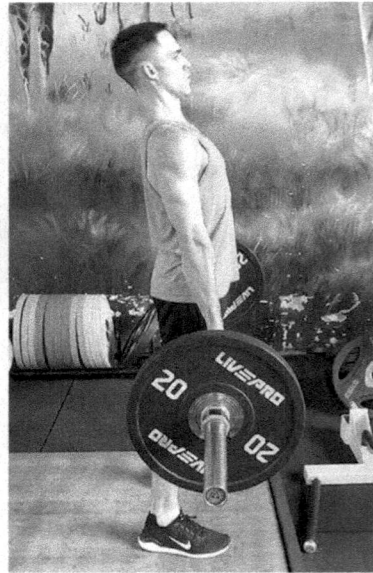

execution:

If you want to try it, I suggest modifying our gym math from earlier. After starting with a low weight, say 80 to 100 pounds total, think about how much weight you could do for 6-10 reps, and then either reduce that weight by 30% or cut your estimated reps in half.

I've personally only been deadlifting for 11 weeks, and my set is 245 pounds for 7 repetitions. The first rep is always the funkiest as you get the weight off the ground while keeping your back straight, then it's a little less awkward. It's also satisfying to drop the bar on the ground after your last repetition, but not all gyms are OK with this behavior. In the example above, I'm on a raised platform intended for deadlifting, and dropping the bar is allowed.

To give deadlifting a try without as many lower back concerns, see if your gym has a trap bar.

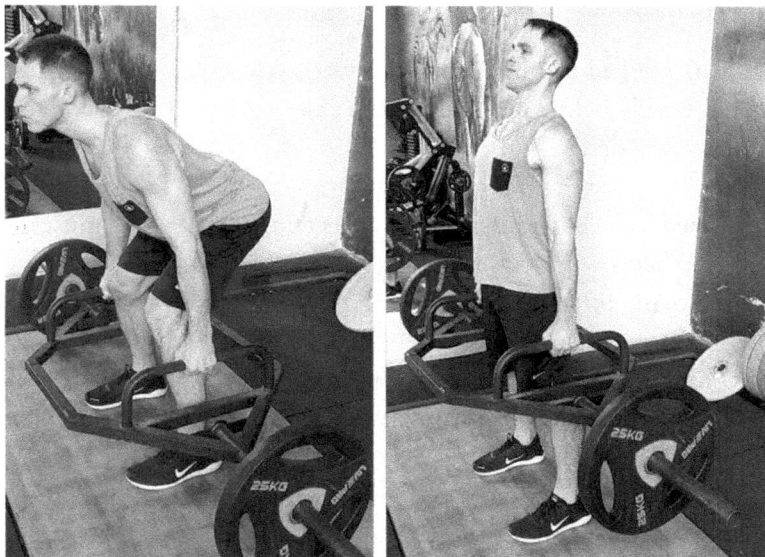

I personally prefer this device because it makes the initial movement of lifting the weight off the floor less awkward. By awkward, I mean: your lower back gets a vulnerable funny feeling, like it's going to "give out."

notes:

I'm making this lift optional for two reasons: it's dangerous if done incorrectly, and it's not practical for most fitness goals. Men have a tendency to overexert themselves at the gym to look tough, which makes weak souls injury-prone.

Because you are not reading Hospital for Hackers, we're going to value our personal instincts above deadlifting. If it feels weird, don't do it. Alternatively, try a much lower weight for several A-Day workouts until your confidence is lifted.

B-DAY BENCHMARKS

If you haven't worked out in a while (or ever), you're likely already sore from capturing A-Day benchmarks. If that's the case, wait a day or two before measuring B-Day lifts described next.

As I mentioned, our A- and B-day workouts converge in some muscle groups but also have their own focus areas. Let's capture benchmarks for a few more lifts before moving on to Chapter 5, The 12 Hour Fitness Experiment.

The first 3 lifts in our B-Day sequence are duplicates from A-Day. Since these muscles are more visually noticeable, we want to more aggressively develop them.

1. bicep curls
2. dips
3. tricep press down

Developing our upper body, particularly arm muscles, is one of the best ways to spot gains sooner than later. Other people in your life will notice too, further fueling your motivation to continue hacking in the gym.

Next, are the new workouts for our B-Day, which are again summarized in text, image, and video at fitnessforhackers.com/videos.

CHIN-UPS

muscles: biceps, shoulders

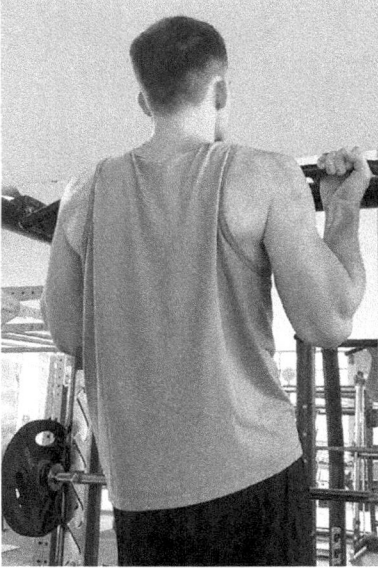

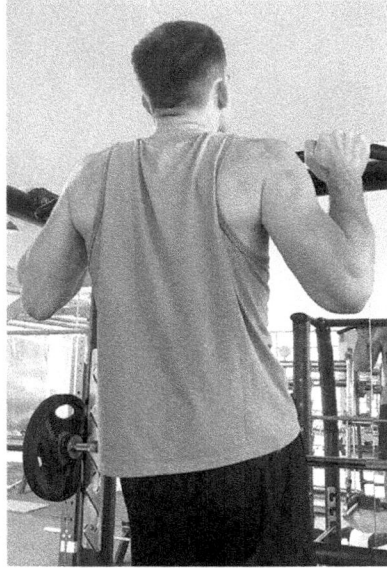

In this illustration, I'm doing a chin-up on the left and a pull up on the right. chin-ups primarily work your biceps, while pull-ups work your lats (upper back).

execution:
Chin-ups and pull-ups are different workouts, but you can decide which one is best for your goals.

A pull up is when your palms face away from you, and usually, you grip the bar at slightly wider points than your shoulders. A chin-up, which in my opinion is easier for beginners, means palms face toward you, and your grip is slightly less wide than your shoulders.

notes:
Chin-ups are another lift that vary greatly in difficulty based on your form. For example, if you cross your feet and pull up slowly, you'll likely be exhausted after just a few (under 10). If you use your own body's momentum and don't lower your-

self all the way between each repetition, you can likely do 10+ on your first try.

While benchmarking your chin-up set, be honest with yourself and aim for slow and full motion vs. a vanity metric.

DUMBBELL SHRUGS

muscles:
trapezius (high back muscles)

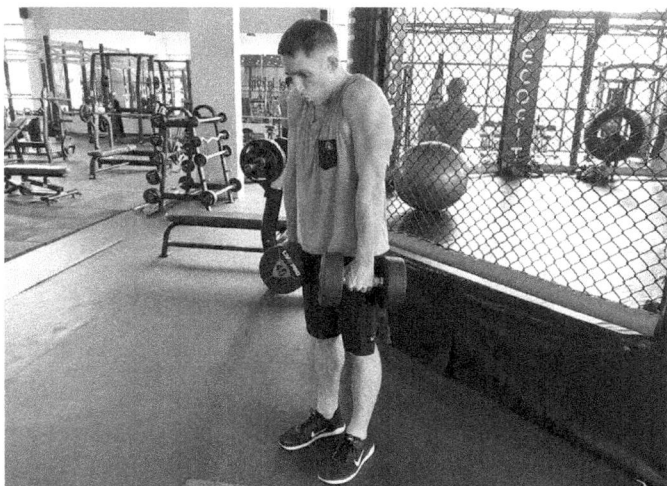

In this illustration, I'm shrugging 40 kilograms per arm, even though I only curl 20 kilograms (45 pounds) per arm. After standing upright, I like to shrug the weight from my back to my front, then reverse, toggling between directions for each repetition in my set.

execution:
Start by lifting the weight off the ground or a nearby bench. Just like deadlifting, keep your back generally straight to prevent injury. You will likely be able to shrug a lot more weight than you can bicep curl, so keep in mind the approach to your initial liftoff is different.

Lift your shoulders as close to your ears as possible and lower the weight in a circular motion toward your knees or your back.

notes:
So far we've done very little to develop our shoulders. On B-Day, we have a few lifts to assist with this, and the first is dumbbell shrugs.

CALF RAISES

muscles:
gastrocnemius, tibialis posterior and soleus muscles (aka lower leg, aka calf)

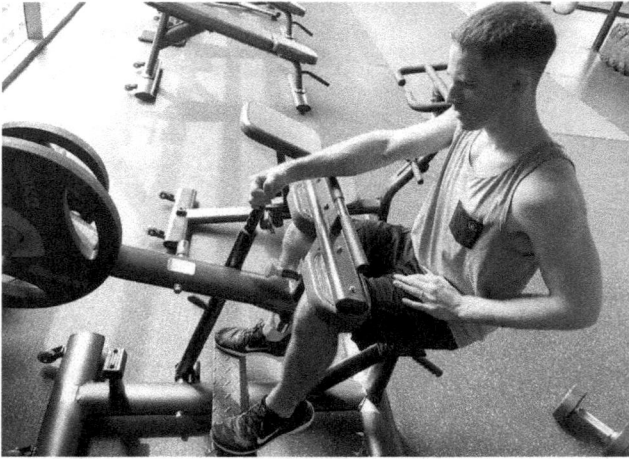

execution:
Using either a calf machine or while simply standing on a ledge with your heels closer to the ground than your toes, simulate "standing on your tippy toes" which in turn will either raise the [plate] weights or your own body weight into the air.

notes:
I'm tempted to make this workout optional, but I hate seeing guys at the gym with "big chests and chicken legs," so the workout lives on.

Because the calves are not accustomed to high resistance or isolated stress (except in the gym), you might leave your first couple B-Day workouts with a bit of a limp and later that night, soreness. This is OK.

What you want to avoid, however, is lifting *too much* weight on your calves.

Instead of soreness, you'll feel a sensation of "permanently flexed muscles," which is seriously uncomfortable and in my experience, it makes it difficult to sleep. Overworking your calves is essentially on-demand RLS (restless leg syndrome).

SQUATS

muscles:
quadriceps (quads), glutes (butt), hamstrings, calves

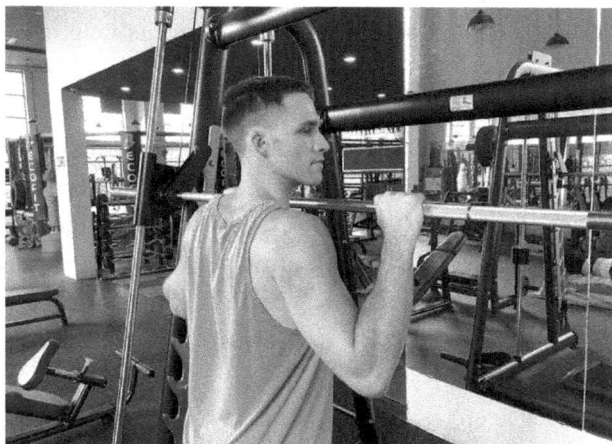

execution:
I can't tell you how many times I started adding plates to the bar and then realized it was set up by a much shorter person.

If you make this mistake, you may be tempted to "muscle up" the weight to a higher rung on the rack, but I don't recommend it. Take off all the plates and reset the bar to your optimal height, then add weights.

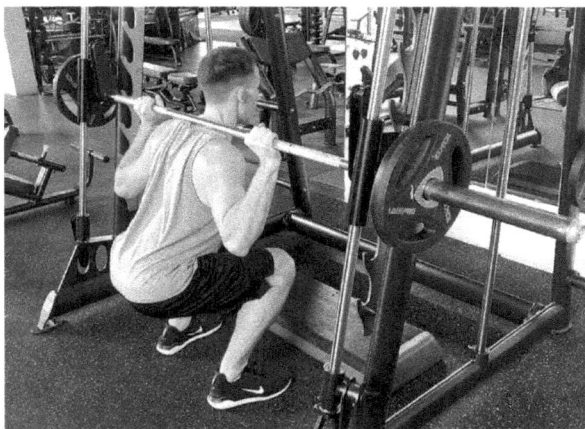

Just like our other lifts, remember that the bar itself weighs around 45 pounds, and if this is your first time squatting, try adding just 10-20 pounds on each side to see how it feels.

Imagine you're doing a "wall sit" and crouch down until your hips are parallel with the floor. Your feet should be about shoulder length apart, but you can spread them wider if it helps you stay balanced.

notes:
Another butt and leg exercise, squats help you with "fun" stuff like playing basketball (jumping) and running (starting speed and acceleration).

You may use either an assisted squat rack, which has "claws" to prevent hurting yourself or a standard squat rack. I prefer the assisted machine because, just like the chest press, it can be dangerous lifting to failure alone.

Before adding any weight to the bar, make sure its height is aligned with the bottom of your neck.

As of this writing, I only squat 215 pounds for 10 repetitions, yet in a high school weight training class my personal best was around 250 pounds. Start small and work your way up.

Some squat machines feature cylinder pads you can wrap around the bar to protect your neck. I'm supportive of these, but know that your neck will get used to the slight discomfort, and a lack of padding should not be a deal-breaker when it's squat (B-) day.

DUMBBELL LATERAL RAISE

muscles:
anterior deltoid, trapezius

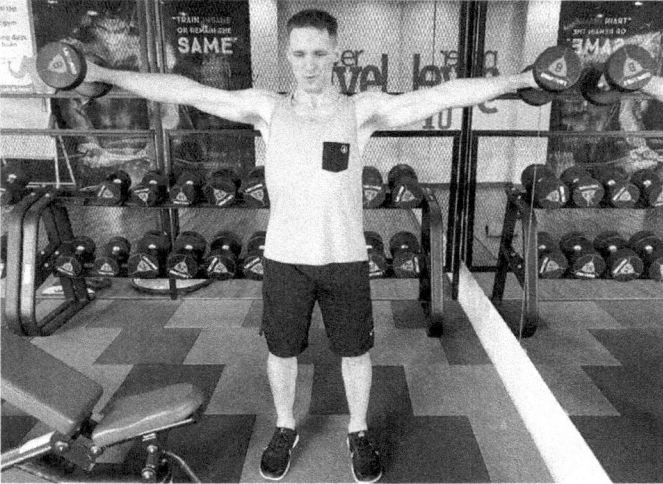

Here I'm raising 8 kilograms (17.5 pounds) to prevent blurry photos.

execution:
Hold dumbbells by your sides, touching your pockets. With your arms locked at the elbows, raise the dumbbells until your arms are slightly beyond being parallel with the floor.

notes:
This lift is one of the most humbling and challenging in our plan. It's also how you'll develop impressive "balled" shoulders to complement your new biceps and triceps.

While I've personally experienced 2-4 gains per week across my A- and B-day sequences, my dumbbell lateral raise has plateaued for several weeks at just 22.5 pounds, 10 repetitions per arm.

It's very difficult to hold your max weight for more than a moment, so develop a smooth cadence of lifting up above your shoulder height, then lower the dumbbells back down toward your hips.

MILITARY PRESS

muscles:
shoulders, triceps

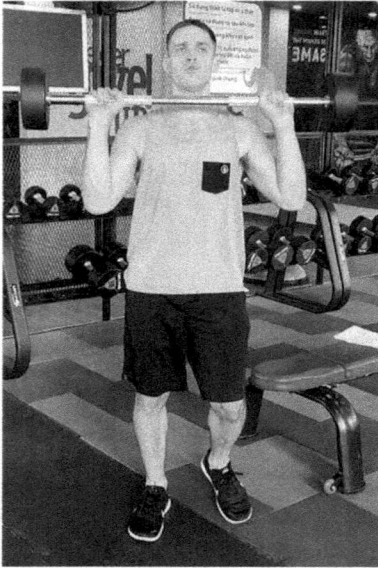

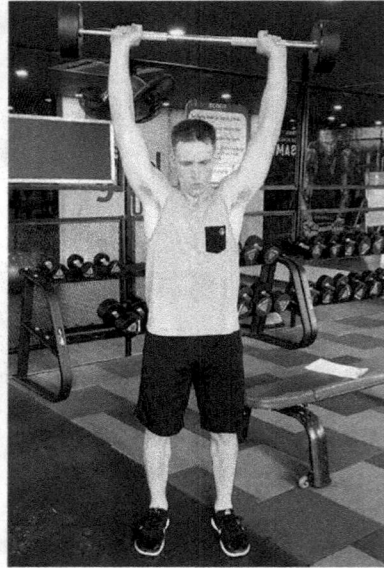

In this illustration, you can see I've taken a step back to balance myself during that initial movement, but after the first repetition, my feet remain planted in one spot.

execution:
I've watched many professional lifters do this press their own way. Froning sticks his head in front of the bar after its raised, positioning the weight just behind his shoulders, and his arms angled slightly backward.

My preferred way to prepare for this lift is by deadlifting the barbell, then bicep curling it toward my chest, and finally flipping my palms to face outward before beginning the first repetition.

notes:
I was inspired to get better at this lift after watching the documentary *"Froning: The Fittest Man in History."* it's about Chris Froning, the only person as of this writing to win the annual CrossFit games 4 times.

In 2014, he presses 245 pounds above his head like it's nothing. For reference, I currently press 110 lbs, 12 times, on my B-Day sequence.

LEG EXTENSION (OPTIONAL)

muscles:

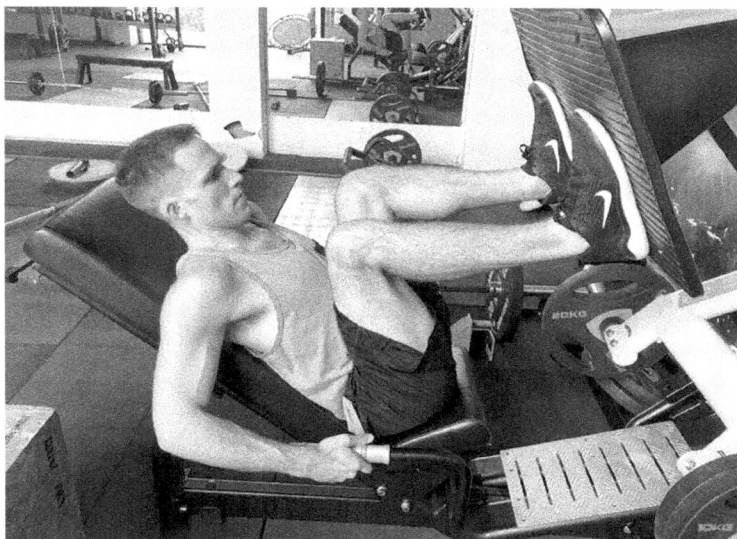

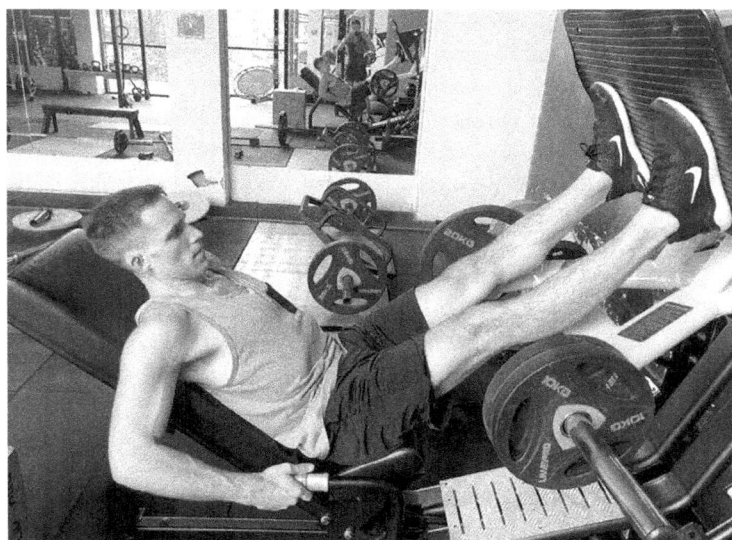

execution:

Weight plates may be added to any of the 2-4 protruding bars, and they're held in place by either a forward / backward lever (depicted here) or a sideways turning beam, usually located right beside your butt.

For most men near my size (5 feet 11 inches), I suggest starting at around 150 pounds to see how that feels. Our optimal set for all these lifts is just 6-10 repetitions. However, I've been breaking that rule as my local gym has a fixed "cable" machine that does not support more than 350 pounds.

Before adding weight, adjust the leg extension machine such that your legs are mostly curled up, and your knees are close to your chest.

Before pressing your legs out for the first repetition, double-check your ability to swiftly switch the weight lock back into position. If your legs ever feel like they're about to buckle, and you haven't studied the machine… you might be in trouble.

notes:

Similar to deadlifting, leg extension (also called leg press) is optional because strong quads aren't a critical feature most of us are looking for.

Further, quads are a complementary muscle to your hamstrings, the muscles on the other (under) side of your upper leg. When you see a professional runner "pull their hamstrings," it's usually due to an inefficient muscle ratio between their quadriceps and hamstrings.

In other words, if you want to work out your quads, it's also a good (safe) idea to do leg curls, but that exercise is not part of this workout plan.

SHIPPING YOUR BENCHMARKS

The measurement process outlined in this chapter should take you about 1 hour to complete in the gym.

Your Trello board should have a card for each of the 15 unique workouts across your A- and B-day sequences. Here's another link to our Fitness template shared first in Chapter 3.

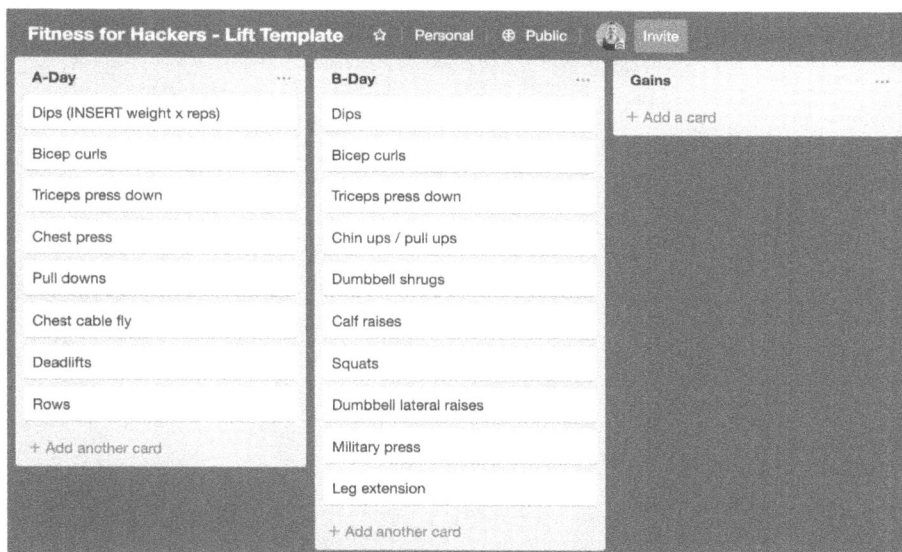

Fitness for Hackers - Lift Template ☆ Personal ⊕ Public Invite		
A-Day ···	**B-Day** ···	**Gains** ···
Dips (INSERT weight x reps)	Dips	+ Add a card
Bicep curls	Bicep curls	
Triceps press down	Triceps press down	
Chest press	Chin ups / pull ups	
Pull downs	Dumbbell shrugs	
Chest cable fly	Calf raises	
Deadlifts	Squats	
Rows	Dumbbell lateral raises	
+ Add another card	Military press	
	Leg extension	
	+ Add another card	

Remember to also insert your weight and reps following our convention:

```
{{ muscle }} {{ lift }} ({{ weight }} x {{ repetitions }})
```

This becomes "Bicep curl (75x8)" on the top left card in your Trello board.

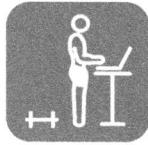

CHAPTER 5

THE 12 HOUR FITNESS EXPERIMENT

"It is a shame for a man to grow old without seeing the beauty and strength of which his body is capable."
— Socrates

You're now halfway through the book and 100% ready to get ripped.

Hackers pride themselves in doing their best work, no matter what the job is. As knowledge workers, the fruits of our labor are cash and status. By extending this work ethic to our physical fitness, we'll reap new benefits through health and looks.

In this chapter, I'm going to outline the 12-hour fitness experiment. This name is not a gimmick—you will literally spend about 1 hour per week in the gym over the next 12 weeks.

Here's that 12-week assignment in 3 parts.

PART 1 - DIET AND FAST

Don't eat crap, and skip breakfast. Repeat after me: breakfast is for losers.

It will be extremely hard to resist a free slice of pizza at work, or donut, or cookie from your pantry. But remember: everyone else, whose body you don't want, eats that stuff. You do not want to be them, so you don't eat like them.

Pending your ability to process carbohydrates and the diet plan you choose from Chapter 2, giving up bread and sugar will probably be the most difficult aspect of your next 12-week journey. Eating fewer calories (if necessary) and spending minimal time in the gym takes a fraction of the brainpower required to restrict shoveling crap in your mouth.

Using the worksheet you copied earlier, set a calorie goal and diary each meal in your tracker tool of choice. I usually log into MyFitnessPal just 1x per day and knock out my lunch and dinner in < 30 seconds. Some mornings I even plan my meals by plugging in a chicken salad for lunch, steak for dinner, by 10am. If it's a rest day from the gym I'm now done with all my apps for 36-48 hours. Easy.

In Chapter 7 on troubleshooting, I'll share a handful of techniques and mental models with which to improve your mental toughness when it comes to eating bad foods.

PART 2 - GYM

Do not ignore the workout plan in Chapter 4. If you hate weights and think "I'll just run" or hate lifting to failure and think "I'll just do 2-3 sets of lower intensity," you will not get the results I know are possible in just 12 weeks. Suck it up.

Here are a few things you can expect over the next 12 weeks of working out:

- extreme resistance: rainy weather; busy days at work with extra-long hours; fatigue
- laziness: working out on weekends, or whatever days you usually relax, will be annoying and feel unfair

- helplessness: if you weigh yourself too often, you'll be "fat" some days and want to give up

Chapters 6 and 7 will touch on more of these challenges and exactly how to address them. But since you're in a positive mindset right now, just acknowledge sometimes it will SUCK to work out, and that's OK.

THE 12-HOUR FITNESS EXPERIMENT EXPLAINED

The name of this chapter is not a gimmick, it's simple math: go to the gym 2x per week, toggling between your A- and B-day sequences, and spend no more than 30 minutes on your lifts. With just 7-10 lifts per session and 1 set per lift, you'll spend no more than 12 hours in the gym over the next 12 weeks.

Since most people spend a lot longer in the gym, cheating themselves with low-intensity workouts and long text message breaks, you might observe a few strange looks from other gym regulars as you move swiftly from machine to machine.

For the overachievers reading this I've outlined *optional* addendums in Chapter 8 that will increase the length of your workouts, and even increase your weekly workout sessions from 2 to 3, but I strongly recommend against incorporating them into your first 12-week regimen.

If you think you'll be tempted to overachieve, simply restart the 12 hour experiment on Week 11 with the extensions outlined in Chapter 8. More on that later.

PART 3 - TRACK

We covered several variables you want to be hyper-aware of during this training experiment. From weight to muscle size, to advanced metrics like your level of ketones and BMI, put in the effort to record your gains and changes over time.

To maintain motivation and turn "fitness kicks" into habits, you need to know your numbers. Entrepreneurs who hate accounting have to know their numbers. Hackers who want to get ripped have to know their numbers too.

1. weigh yourself 1x /week, around the same time and context (I weigh-in Sunday mornings before lunch)
2. measure your body parts 1x week, preferably during your weigh-in
3. be honest about what you're eating and record it to understand weekly weight changes

While tracking your food intake, workouts, and body composition changes don't directly impact your overall health, it does influence your thoughtfulness in following through.

Believe it or not, the tracking component actually has the capacity to *destroy your entire experiment* if not taken seriously. Here's one realistic way it can play out, which I'm sharing so you can avoid.

First you forget to track 1, 2, or 3 meals in a row. Each time you miss, you mentally "log" what you ate so you can plug it in later. Maybe you don't have WiFi, are in a movie theater, whatever. Only then, you have a questionable meal or snack. Either something you shouldn't eat (donut), or can't easily break down into simple ingredients (General Tso Chicken). You know that logging this will jack up your [otherwise good] numbers, so you lie to yourself and go to sleep. The next day you feel sluggish and skip your scheduled work-out: "*I'll catch up tomorrow.*" another couple days go by, and you now owe yourself 7-10 meals in your tracker, 2 workouts + gains in your Trello, and a weigh-in that you know won't be pretty because you're constipated on General Tso and Donuts from the networking event.

At this point, you're only 7 days into our 12-hour experiment and already back to Fat Hacker status. You're pissed! And it's all because you didn't thumb tap your calorie tracker.

I'll let you in on a secret: the revenue from this book that I keep will be from low-energy readers who don't heed this advice. By including this all-too-real scenario, it is my goal to make $0 from the book and instead see 1,000s of ripped hackers in the fitnessforhackers.com community.

TIME COMMITMENTS AT THE GYM

If you aren't used to training in a gym, your first few visits may take a bit longer than the 30 minutes I've promised.

I suggest opening up Chapter 4 on your phone and methodically moving from lift to lift, toggling between the book illustrations and your Trello board to commit the workouts to memory.

As you practice each lift without assistance from the book, you'll eventually only need Trello for gains and lift organization. Personally, I like to rearrange the ordering of my lifts, and this is almost necessary as you may find another gym rat is already using the machine you want. No sweat, just drag and drop another Trello card up your list and do that lift first.

MEASURING GAINS THE EASY WAY

I know there are a lot of fitness tracker apps, and half of you reading this could probably build your own over a weekend.

But we're aiming for efficiency, and no single tracker will make all readers happy. If I endorse one, others will complain, and Fitness for Hackers is not a product review resource. We're interested in what works, what is efficient, and what is already familiar to readers. Kanban for lifts, spreadsheets for metrics, and loggers for calories do the job.

For now, here's how to visualize your gains over time:

1. complete a given lift, i.e. "Biceps 60 pounds x 8 reps," with more reps (say 10 instead of 8)
2. duplicate the "Bicep curls" card in your Trello board
3. move the duplicated card to the very top of your far-right list, titled "Gains"
4. change the title of the original Bicep curls card to reflect your gain, i.e. "Bicep curls (60x10)"
5. you're done

Your Gains list is now a reverse-chronologically sorted history of every lift (weight and repetitions) you've conquered in your journey. Likewise, the original Trello card for a given lift has full history as well.

Clicking open a specific lift card on your phone will look like this:

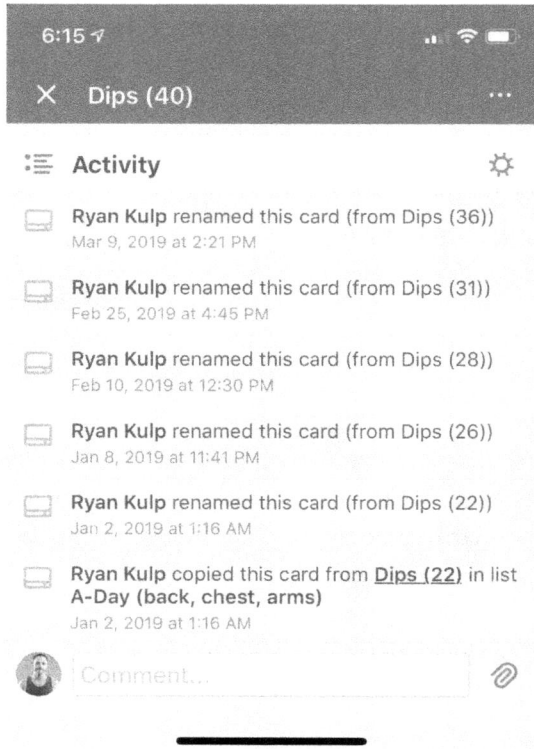

You not only know where you started with a given lift, but how often you clocked a gain and what the difference was. Sometimes high tech solutions look a lot like low tech tools.

My personal goal is to experience 1-3 gains per week, and it's all tracked in the poor man's fitness planner.

GYM JARGON

In Chapter 4, we introduced a handful of terms that may not have sunk in yet if you're new to the gym.

Here are those concepts again:

- isolated lifts—movements that primarily work out 1 muscle in your body. We prefer these over compound lifts because they let us focus on building each muscle to be as strong as it can be at its own pace.
- compound lifts—motions like kettlebell swings and even deadlifts that develop multiple muscles during the repetition.
- lift to failure—a popular weight lifting strategy we subscribe to at Fitness for Hackers, which suggests you should build muscle by completing 1 set of a given lift vs. 2-3 sets with lower weights. While sometimes uncomfortable, this is more efficient and sustainable for hackers who don't want to live in the gym.
- repetition—a single movement of a given lift.
- set—a group of repetitions done back to back.
- resistance—often a synonym for "weight," but some machines use arbitrary values, especially cycling and stair stepper cardio machines.
- barbell—wide (5 feet / 1 meter or longer) or narrow (3 feet / 1 meter) bars. Can have predefined weights or be "naked" and allow any number of plates to be added on either end.
- dumbbell—hand-held weights, like miniature barbells. Can be substituted for barbell style workouts but generally require more discipline to use correctly, as they cause wobbly left / right side muscle movements.

- weight collars—circular "belts," usually just 3-4 inches wide, that can be locked around the outside of a plate to prevent it from sliding off. Especially useful for squats, deadlifts, and bench press.
- free weights—barbells and dumbbells, plates and racks. "Hardcore" lifters swear by free weights but we're more interested in safety and efficiency, so free weights are just one option to us.
- assisted / machines—accomplish the same stress on our muscles as free weights, sometimes even more so as they prevent overcompensation from either side of our body. Helpful for lift to failure style workouts due to built-in protections and guard rails.
- bench—any narrow "chair" or padding. Most can be modified to lay flat, inclined, or declined. Used for bench press as well as alternative workouts such as dips without a dip machine.
- platform—not available in all gyms, but usually intended for deadlift and squat workouts that end in dropping a bar on the floor.
- swinging—when you get clever with momentum and use existing bodyweight to "assist" in a lift.

As we explore advanced techniques and workouts in Chapter 8, we'll make those additional key terms and concepts available for reference at fitnessforhackers.com.

PRESS GO

If you haven't already:

1. spend 1-2 days at the gym this week to benchmark your max weight and repetitions for 15 single-set lifts
2. measure your body and record the results in your **Fitness for Hackers worksheet** introduced in Chapter 3
3. log your meals in a calorie tracker app

Once this is done, move on to Chapter 6.

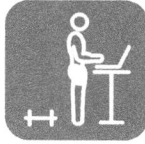

CHAPTER 6

CREATING MULTIPLE POINTS OF FAILURE

"The more you sweat in training, the less you bleed in combat."
— Richard Marcinko

In software development, a single point of failure (called SPoF) is a component in a system that breaks everything if it fails. In other words, SPoF-fractured systems are fragile as they lack the flexibility to accommodate mistakes.

The solution to SPoF architecture is redundancy: backup routes that handle the load when a peer component breaks. Redundant systems are therefore more robust, but also the most expensive to maintain. Early stage products are littered with SPoF, and "fitness kick" workout plans are too.

At Fitness for Hackers, we avoid SPoF by equipping ourselves with a contingency plan to every part of our routine, from tracking meals to fasting to lifting weights in the gym. The following are common SPoF scenarios you'll encounter as you work Fitness for Hackers into your schedule.

Some are purely circumstantial, a reflection of life as we know it: unpredictable, Murphy's Law[10], busy schedules. Some other points of failure are more insidious. Steven Pressfield describes this second group well in his bestseller *The War of Art,* aptly branding it *resistance:*[11]

> *"Resistance, by definition, is self-sabotage. But there's a parallel peril that must also be guarded against: sabotage by others.*
>
> *When a writer begins to overcome her Resistance… she may find that those close to her begin acting strange… they may accuse the awakening writer of 'changing,' of 'not being the person she was.'*
>
> *… they are trying to sabotage her."*

FRIENDS, FAMILY, AND COLLEAGUES

When you begin to eat right and exercise, at least 1 person in your life will resist your decision.

This may sound counter-intuitive and dramatic, especially if you love your friends and coworkers, but it's a subconscious reaction and out of your control.

Perhaps one of your colleagues tried and failed to lose weight, or at least to stop eating free donuts at networking events. When they notice you resisting crap food successfully, they'll come up with excuses to rationalize why it's "easier for you" or, more damaging, they'll vocalize these grievances to taunt you back into their sluggish, unremarkable lifestyle.

I'm no cartoon guy, but Disney's rendition of *Hercules* has a scene that captures this sentiment precisely.[12]

Hercules has just dived into the Underworld to save Meg. A colony of dead souls tugs to hold him down while The Fates attempt to cut his "life thread." they almost succeed, except his selfless sacrifice renders him immortal, affording him the time to climb out of the sea of dead souls. Then Hades, who initially tricked him into this suicide rescue mission, is himself dragged into the Underworld by those same dead spirits who endeavor nothing more than to be accompanied in eternal misery.

Some of the people in your life are like those dead souls. They've given up on their personal fitness aspirations, and to mitigate their dissatisfaction, they will attempt to pull you down to their level in the midst of your ascension. They will offer free pizza, cookies, a Corona. They will tease you with feel-good phrases like *"come on, live a little."*

But you've already lived a little. You lived a LOT. And now you're reading this book to live even better.

At first, their resistance might be playful and well-intentioned. If the teasing continues past the point of laughter, however, you need to acknowledge *they are projecting personal insecurities*. It is not your job to fix this unless you are their therapist.

ALCOHOL

To be fair to our friends, they aren't the only reason we put poison in our bodies. Geography also plays a part.

When I packed my bags and left New York City, a place well known for drinking culture, my alcohol consumption dropped almost to zero simply by placing myself outside the zip code of drinking buddies. Fast forward a couple weeks, I reversed my other bad habit of ordering cocktails at nice restaurant dinners and boom: I'm liquor-free.

Cutting out alcohol alone can yield 1+ pounds lost per week without any other changes to your diet or behavior. While we advocate a comprehensive program to maximize results, keep in mind that even a few hundred calories saved per day adds up to material changes in your body composition, gym exercise aside. Remember: do not drink calories.

In hacker fashion, next are visualized if-given-when procedures for navigating common points of failure that will arise in your fitness journey.

MISSING A WORKOUT

First off, schedule your workouts.

We only need 2 per week to get in great shape, so there's no reason to "play it by ear." I like to keep my weekends open for sleeping in, working on side projects, and exploring, so this means I work out Monday / Thursday or Tuesday / Friday. Setting a schedule removes all processing power required to get your butt in the gym.

Nevertheless, sometimes you'll miss a scheduled workout.

- you exercise after work, but have a company dinner / event / stayed late at the office
- you exercise before work but have a networking breakfast / up late the night before / dropping off kids
- it's time to work out, and you just don't feel like it

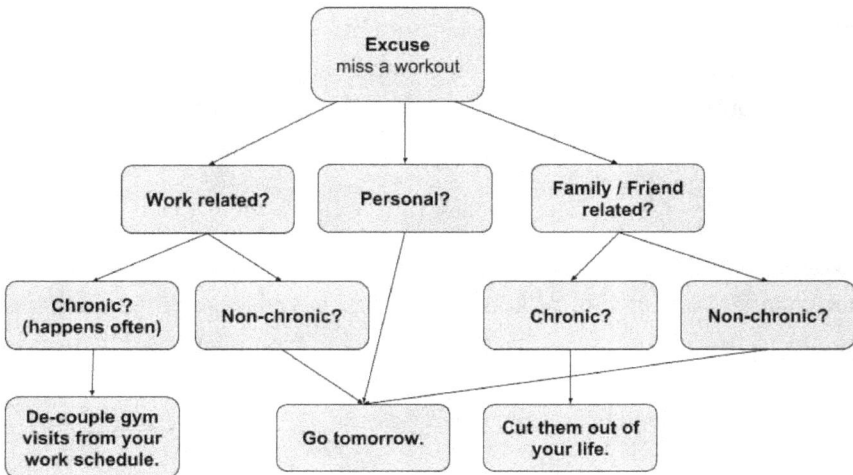

Missing workouts is the beginning of the end for the entire Fitness for Hackers regimen. If you forget to track a meal, but ate well, or forget to record a fast, but skipped breakfast, this is redeemable because you still did The Work.

Not exercising, however, kicks off a downward spiral back to fatness and a shorter lifespan with fewer complements.

Be vigilant in making your workouts, even when it hurts. More on that in the next two flowcharts.

YOUR GYM SUCKS

Whether you rely on a crummy apartment gym or travel a lot like I do, you may not have all the tools you need to hit each of your lifts on a 2x /weekly basis.

In Chapter 5, I covered a few alternatives for this scenario, including:

- partial-body dips using a bench or other raised platform, like a chair. Multiply your max count by 1.5.
- standing rows with free weights (dumbbells) at a lower weight and 2x-3x repetitions.

But there's more. Instead of weighted squats, do air squats. This is the same motion as a weighted squat but without the bar. If your usual set is 7-10 squats with 100 pounds, try 3 sets of 25 squats with your empty palms facing the ceiling.

As for chin-ups, you can usually find an apparatus on which to do these wherever you are. Sometimes a sturdy door frame will work, otherwise, try standing underneath a short stairwell and gripping the floor beside the railing of the level above.

Do jumping jacks instead of dumbbell lateral raises. Stand tippy toe on a curb or stair for "organic calf raises." and instead of bench press, do pushups.

Sometimes while traveling, I'm forced to do a home workout. Here's my full routine, which takes about 15 minutes:

1. air squats - 20 repetitions
2. pushups - 20 repetitions
3. crunches - 20 repetitions

After 5-10 seconds of rest, I repeat this sequence 6 to 8 times. If short on time or I've procrastinated my workout all day, I opt for "jumping" pushups prior to hopping in the shower at night.

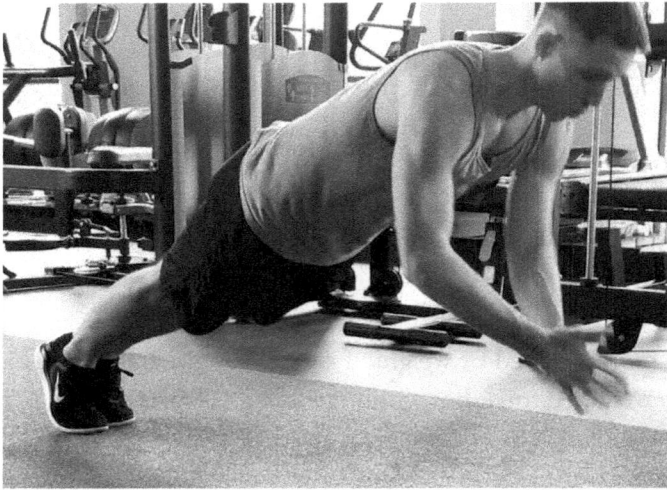

In this variation, you push yourself off the ground with enough force that you can clap your hands together before your body falls back toward the floor.

If working out is a new element in your lifestyle, don't worry if you can't hack these on your first try. I waited until I could do over 120 pushups in 3 minutes before practicing this style, and I'm still not very good at it.

Ultimately, jumping pushups are just a slightly more efficient way to work out your chest. They're also kind of fun. After 1-2 sets of 10 or 20, I'm done for the day, and it's time to shower.

LOSS OF STRENGTH

Not all workouts are created equal.

Sometimes you'll hit the gym and feel sluggish. Maybe you didn't get enough sleep or have a bad attitude, or aren't focused on the task at hand. As a result, you'll find that each of your workouts feels "harder," like you set an unrealistic repetition count or weight amount in a previous, more optimistic session.

Luckily, workouts under these conditions can be salvaged, and you can still build muscle vs. merely maintain, even on the bad days.

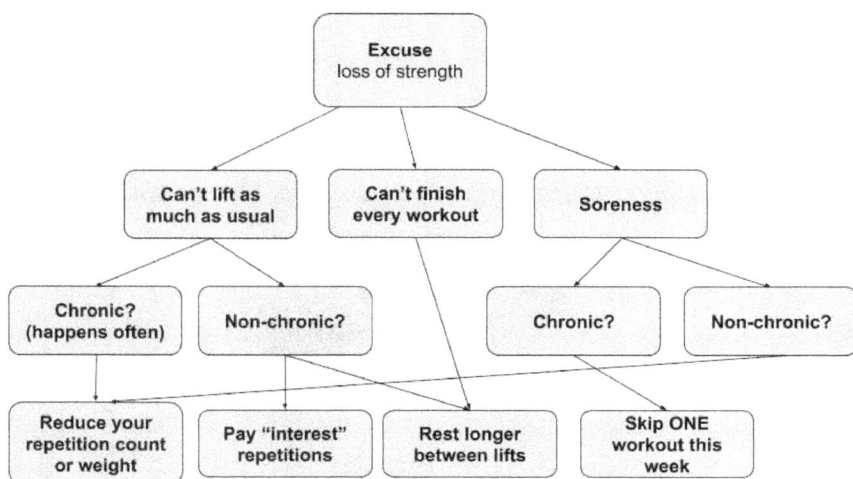

Technical debt happens when we write poor code that has to be rewritten later, often at a greater cost. Most software teams create technical debt on a weekly basis, as business goals often compel the need for speed over quality. This is OK within reason, and our term for "paying back" technical debt is Interest.

Sometimes we'll experience technical debt in our fitness plans, and that too needs to be paid back with Interest.

If you find, for example, that you're unable to lift your usual weight of 100 pounds, 6 times straight, compete your workout in 2 sets of 4 and 3. The second set of 3 repetitions (instead of 2) represents 1 "interest repetition" over your intended max repetition count.

By paying interest on workouts that fall short of our established goals, two things happen:

1. you get better at setting weight and repetition benchmarks
2. you learn to "suck it up" during a given workout and finish your single set in one swoop

CARDIO SUBSTITUTE

Some days you might daydream about running or sitting on a bike instead of the usual lift to failure strategy that is paramount to the Fitness for Hackers regimen.

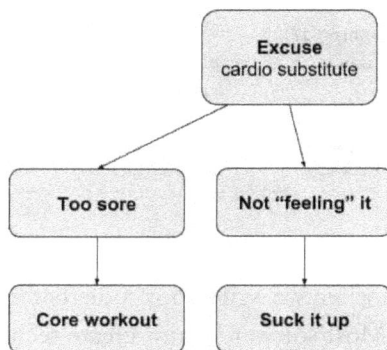

I predict most of these days you're just facing The Resistance.

Maybe you weighed in the day before and gained 5 pounds since last week. Maybe you scarfed General Tso [fried, breaded] chicken last night at your cousin Bobby's Superbowl party (his roommate makes good queso) and are kicking yourself with defeatist *"what's the point?"* self talk.

Regardless of your Why, practice adapting by *leaning into* the pain.

Recently I looked in the mirror and noticed my teeth were markedly yellow, more than usual. Since I've been away from home the last few months, I typically work out of cafes and drinking coffee all day without enough water or teeth brushing in between explains this discoloration.

So I booked a laser teeth whitening session.

At first, it went well... the hygienist did a routine teeth cleaning to prepare me for the treatment, then gave me some anesthetic and off we went, laser to mouth for 4, fifteen-minute sessions.

By the middle of the second session, my mouth was on fire. The best description I can offer is it felt like my teeth were hooked up to an electric shock machine. Every 10 to 20 seconds, a "wave" of electricity, which I later learned was a typical "enamel sensitivity reaction," overcame my mouth, and all I could do was *wince*. I couldn't move because the laser was strapped to my face.

After a few rounds of this self-induced torture, I began to cultivate the pain. I tried to visualize it hitting my molars in the back of my mouth instead of my front teeth, where the sensation was most uncomfortable. And it began to work.

While the pain didn't suck any less, and it lasted another several hours after the procedure, I was still able to read a chapter of a research paper, try new restaurants for lunch and dinner, and get some work done on this book.

This is what sucking it up looks like, and it's a superpower you'll need to foster in order to conquer the 12-hour experiment prescribed in Fitness for Hackers.

As for the days when you simply feel too sore and think cardio is a rational alternative, instead, plot out a C-Day in your A/B sequence that consists primarily of core workouts:

- torso curl
- suspended leg raises
- weighted decline crunches

I'll discuss these again in Chapter 8, but for now, just know that you don't have to injure yourself for the sake of sticking to our schedule. There is always a backup plan because we've built redundancy directly into our fitness program.

WORKING OUT AFTER A BIG MEAL

Sometimes the best medicine is preventive.

In other words, it's best to schedule workouts *before* meals and skip this point of failure entirely. You'll feel a lot better eating protein and chugging water if you just clocked a gain than if you eat as a way to procrastinate your gym session.

That said, it happens. Instead of waiting until "your stomach settles" because that's just a more sophisticated brand of procrastination, go directly from your meal to the gym and walk on the treadmill for 15-20 minutes before lifting weights.

You can listen to a podcast or audiobook, or even watch your favorite episode of The Mindy Project if the gym has televisions. Condition yourself to not allow meals to impact your decision to work out.

Along the same wavelength, by the way, you'll learn to appreciate a large (healthy) meal *after* a workout. Modern day consumers have convinced ourselves to "pre-fuel," whereas we should spend the gas we have first, then re-fuel.

JUNK FOOD FOR BAD MOODS

I'll be the first to admit: I'm flawed.

Sometimes I spend all day fighting fires at work, and my natural reaction is to eat chocolate or snack on my wife's supply of dried fruit.

There are a couple ways to mitigate this, and neither includes finding a new job or practicing meditation. While both of those strategies are positive, they're out of scope for this book. Instead, the key is to de-risk your cravings.

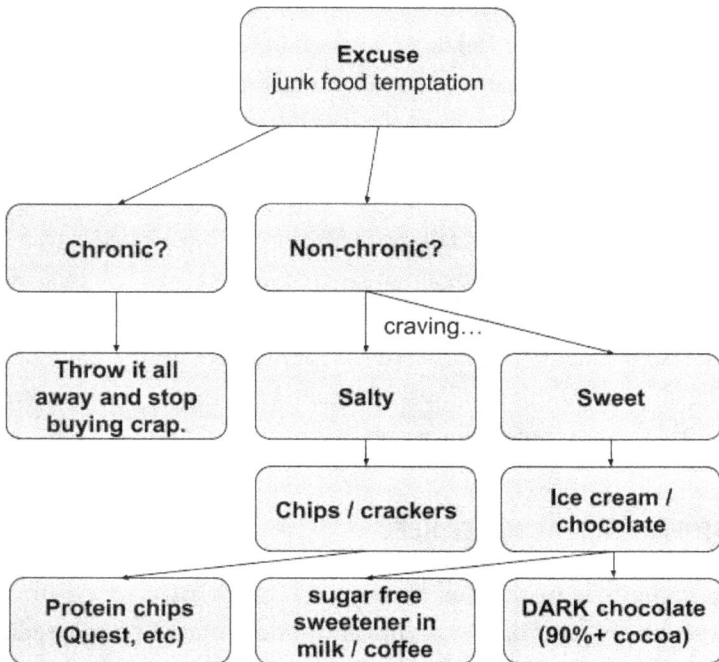

You don't need an ounce of willpower if you don't buy junk in the first place, but many of us live with roommates or a partner, making the contents of our pantry not completely in our control.

For example, my wife snacks all day long and eats every kind of carbohydrate without any effect on her body. It's not uncommon to observe her smacking and crunching chips (she calls them "chipees") late into the evening. It's tough to watch, to be honest, and no, she did not approve this paragraph in my book.

So sometimes I partake. But instead of milk chocolate, I eat dark chocolate. This doesn't taste nearly as good, and by the end of a small piece, I'm already ready to switch back to health mode. In essence, I find the occasional pinch of regret is net-positive for a healthy lifestyle because it reminds us of our Why.

To skip caloric regrets altogether, learn to simulate the future "post-bite" scenario. Imagine breaking a Snickers bar in half, touching your tongue against the salty peanuts and oozing caramel, then logging 229 calories[13] and 30 grams carbohydrates in your food tracker. Was it worth 15 seconds of empty pleasure to negate this morning's workout?

Nonetheless, all of this could fail. Sometimes you have a bad day, get stressed or depressed, and you ran out of sugar-free alternatives. In this case, *reduce your portion*. Instead of taking your roommate's *bag* of chips to the couch, pour some on a small plate. Observe the serving size on the back of the packaging: "12 chips, 340 calories." record this in your logger. If you're still desperate, crush them and prepare for regret.

STRENGTHEN YOUR ACHILLES HEEL

One technique that works well for my own snack avoidance is to brush my teeth immediately after dinner and drink hot tea until I go to sleep. Or, keep drinking coffee (knowing I'll be up until 4am) because this at least has the effect of curbing one's appetite.

The bottom line is: if you're going to screw up, mitigate your losses. I once jokingly said to a ripped guy, "*I could never have a body like yours… I just love Dr. Pepper too much*" (notice the projection of my insecurities, attempting to bring him to my low level).

His reply? "*man I love Dr. Pepper too! that's why sometimes I buy a can of Diet Dr. Pepper, take a huge swig for taste, then spit it out and throw away the can.*"

My almost daily "hack" is to put sugar-free **Torani caramel syrup**[14] in my coffee, sometimes adding almond milk or a few drops of vanilla extract. My wife prefers going to the grocery store and literally "looking" at cakes, then reading the nutritional value labels to remind herself a slice is 500 calories and not worth it. Do what works for you.

EXCEPTION CLASS

Notice that we are not making exceptions to our "no snacking" rule introduced in Chapter 2. At this stage of our diet-only and single-workout experiment, we haven't achieved anything to warrant even the occasional mistake.

In a few days, however, you'll be exercising 2x a week and fasting regularly. You won't be snacking or drinking on a daily basis, and you should be losing 1-2 pounds per week (or more) if that's your goal.

So while Fitness for Hackers does not endorse "cheat days," life happens and these are just a couple ways to optimize for it.

GET FIT FOR FREE

Throughout this book, I've made a handful of refund references to eliminate non-serious spectators. Now I'm making that same offer to you.

While most authors need to get paid for their work, this one is fortunate to depend on software. My writing is about exposing ideas and building a community, not making money.

To prove this, I'm offering a 100% refund if you commit to the following:

1. adopt the Fitness for Hackers challenge for 12 weeks. This includes tracking everything from your intermittent fasts to your meals, body composition to lift gains. You must also train twice per week.
2. send me before and after photos at fitnessforhackers.com/refund to prove you aren't full of crap. As they used to say when I worked at Red Bull: *pics or it didn't happen.*

If your progress photos are legit, I'll refund whatever you paid for the book. I suspect this, in addition to living longer and looking better naked, will motivate you to become your best self.

But we're not done yet.

PART II SUMMARY

By setting public expectations in your immediate ecosystem and becoming hyper-aware of both your current metrics and intended goals, you have the tools you need to make a serious impact on your personal health.

Before moving on:

- hit the gym and establish benchmarks
- let close friends and family members know about your 12-week experiment
- refine your goals and set up all your tracking tools

In Part III, we level up our mindset and behaviors to make Fitness for Hackers, not just a regimen but a lifestyle.

PART II NOTES

1. https://anamaria.martinezgomez.name/2018/12/21/ruby2_6.html
2. https://www.physio-pedia.com/Functional_Movement_Screen_(FMS)
3. https://www.menshealth.com/fitness/a19548367/the-metaconda-workout/
4. referral link: https://amzn.to/2Hbt7hc // non-referral link: https://www.amazon.com/gp/product/B01IF54RKA/
5. referral link: https://amzn.to/2Hdaeu1 // non-referral link: https://www.amazon.com/gp/product/B01MUB7BUV/
6. https://www.builtlean.com/2012/09/24/body-fat-percentage-men-women/
7. https://blog.myfitnesspal.com/8-trainer-approved-ways-to-overcome-gym-anxiety/
8. http://www.nfl.com/news/story/0ap3000000537126/article/football-fit-a-look-at-herschel-walkers-workout-routine
9. inspired by Mark Twain's "I never let my schooling get in the way of my education," https://quoteinvestigator.com/2010/09/25/schooling-vs-education/
10. Murphy's Law: anything that can go wrong, will. https://en.wikipedia.org/wiki/Murphy%27s_law

11. The War of Art, Steven Pressfield: https://www.amazon.com/War-Art-Winning-Creative-Battle/dp/1501260626
12. Hercule vs Hades, https://www.youtube.com/watch?v=Ts_WDlgNMoo
13. Snickers, 1.66oz bar https://ndb.nal.usda.gov/ndb/foods/show/19359
14. Torani Sugar-Free Classic Caramel Syrup with Splenda: https://amzn.to/2XSzATY

PART III

RETENTION

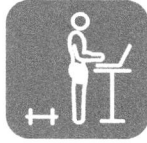

CHAPTER 7

TROUBLESHOOTING

*"I hated every minute of training, but I
said, 'Don't quit. Suffer now and live the
rest of your life as a champion.'"*
— Muhammad Ali

If you have no friends, family, or social responsibilities, the first 6 chapters should get you where you want to go. For the rest of us, there are troubleshooting techniques to help live in harmony with bad influences.

Like Friday morning donuts at the office. Your friend's birthday dinner next weekend. The upcoming family vacation to Italy where seemingly the only options are pasta and pizza.

I've been there, literally. To all of these places and contexts. And I failed hard, too, until I adopted a new mindset.

THERE IS A CONSPIRACY AGAINST YOU

I'm not a conspiracy theorist, but I find them to be useful heuristics for the few among us who care about our bodies and health. My personal favorite: there is a conspiracy against being in good shape. Your colleagues, spouse, even children, all prefer you to be fat and lethargic.

There are good reasons for this, and not so good reasons. Primitively speaking, influencing those around us to be docile reduces predatory threats. Break and enter thieves don't campaign against the police officer special down at Dunkin' Donuts. Concerned citizens do. In short: it's not in our best interest when those around us can easily hurt us.

As for the not so good reason: humans are insecure. Being confronted with a great body, a great mind, a great book, a great competitor's product, forces us to look inward at our inadequacies. It forces us to ask ourselves why we don't have what it takes to be *that*. To do *that*.

When donuts show up at the office, and you turn your nose, expect a colleague to say something like: "come on, just one." or "come on, don't make me feel bad." this is their own insecurity, manifest (disguised?) in playful camaraderie, designed to keep you docile and weak.

Rather than avoid these moments through reclusive behavior, lean into them. Assume there is a conspiracy against your fitness, and everything will start to click.

Your favorite sandwich spot charging extra for "unwich" lettuce over bread? Conspiracy. Half-off, freshly baked cookies at the grocery store checkout? Conspiracy. Saturday night after a long, hard week at work? It's a social construct that weekends are for "damaging our bodies" instead of merely resting. Conspiracy.

IT'S NOT ABOUT WILLPOWER

Author Mark Manson digs deep in behavioral psychology, or why we do what we do. In a blog post on willpower, he says, *"willpower is fleeting... you have to grow to enjoy it."* [1]

A friend of mine, Sam, tells a story about how his mom went on a strict health kick. To force the entire household to conform, she wiped the fridge of all the fun stuff: Coke, cookies, gone. At first, he hated it, but a few months later, in a sermon at our youth church, he shared an insight: *"we don't consume what we crave, we crave what we consume."*

The coconut water and green juice in his diet, at first a nuisance, had become a way of life. His *default*. Our aim in Fitness for Hackers is to create a new default, not supercharge our willpower.

A few years ago, I was reflecting on my skills as a musician. I'm a more talented violinist, yet I spend more time playing guitar. To ease myself back into playing the violin, I didn't force willpower, make calendar reminders, or develop a preference for Tchaikovsky over Drake.

I simply bought a $15 wall hanger and acknowledged the potency of convenience: *you play more when it's out.*

If your workout clothes are in the bottom drawer, your running shoes are in the back of the closet, or your gym itself is the opposite direction from your office or favorite neighborhood, you will go to the gym less often.

HABITS

By now, you've developed thousands of habits. To transition from unhealthy to healthy, less muscle to more muscle, or more fat to less fat, you likely need to break a few habits and make a few more.

Leading habit expert James Clear calls this the Four Laws of Behavior Change in his bestseller *Atomic Habits*.[2]

Form a habit:

1. make it obvious
2. make it attractive
3. make it easy
4. make it satisfying

Break a habit:

1. make it invisible
2. make it unattractive
3. make it difficult
4. make it unsatisfying

To encourage more of the behaviors we want—going to the gym and eating healthy food—we can combine ideas on willpower and convenience into joining a gym that's on our way to work. We can find satisfaction in black coffee (vs. *Frappuccinos*) by adding a bit of Stevia. We can take progress pics every weekend to appreciate changes in our body composition.

These tasks, which require just a few seconds to complete, reinforce the habits that ultimately change our lives. To discourage bad behaviors that destroy our bodies, self-confidence, and lifespan, we can use these laws to achieve the inverse effect on bad behaviors.

Practically speaking, we don't need willpower to avoid eating ice cream. Per Clear's "make it invisible" inversion Law #1, we can simply not buy ice cream. To make sleeping in unattractive and encourage morning gym sessions, we can go to bed with our blinds open. I do this frequently, and it creates a sort of natural alarm system because the sun shines in early and makes falling back asleep almost impossible.

If you find yourself struggling with things like food logging, weekly strength metrics tracking or going to the gym, first ensure you are making each of those routines obvious, attractive, easy, and satisfying. If being fit is inconvenient, it won't stick.

Part of being a hacker is finding the path of least resistance. Your objective, then, is to make fitness congruent with that path.

DIAGNOSTICS

While writing this book, I have spoken with dozens of hackers around the world. I asked each of them: what's your biggest struggle when you try to gain or lose weight?

Here are the top 4 responses, paraphrased:

1. overeating
2. lifestyle
3. consistency at the gym
4. seeing results

overeating

Let's define overeating as consuming 500 or more calories than your BMR (basal metabolic rate) can sustain on a regular basis. If one overeats 5 days per week, a 1-2 pound per week fat loss plan is essentially break-even, destroyed.

The #1 cause of overeating, however, isn't "big meals." it's snacking. Specifically, snacking between dinner and bedtime. Or if your office has a kitchen, snacking between lunch and when you go home.

The single most impactful modification you can implement to curb snacking. Thus, overeating, is intermittent fasting. I personally prefer eating dinner around 7:30p, then fasting 16 hours until noon tomorrow.

On the rare occasion I do snack, I eat pork rinds, beef jerky, cold cuts, and eggs. This could break your fast, but more protein or calories isn't nearly as damaging as carbohydrates or sugar.

Another strategy to avoid overeating is meal prep. This is where you buy or cook a week's worth of food in advance, then quickly warm it up when it's time to eat. Not only are healthy meals now mere moments away from consumption when you get hungry, but you'll be less tempted to spontaneously get fast food. Warning: those who swear by meal prep often spend a few hours in the kitchen every Sunday night. If this sounds like a good time, enjoy.

lifestyle

Remember: there is a conspiracy against you.

Boxers learn early on that you can't avoid (slip) every punch. But you can turn your cheek in the punch's direction. Letting your body move with the punch, vs. resisting, reduces the blow's impact.

How this translates to hacker life: next time you're at a bar, order a tequila soda instead of a beer. Then order just a soda. Fast forward 1 hour, the damage is under 100 calories. And by the way, make sure it's club soda, not tonic, which has 100+ calories alone. You can further reduce the damage by ordering 1 alcoholic beverage, then 1 water with lime, interchangeably.

spirit	calories per shot (1.5oz)[3]
vodka	93
tequila	96
rum	64
gin	110

In my own experience living in heavy drinking cities like Atlanta (4 years), New York City (6 years), and San Francisco (1 year), it's natural to think *"well, I'm at a bar, guess I have to cheat."* we succumb to the conspiracy. But this is a lie because there are alternatives, so stop lying to yourself.

When you can't avoid the punch altogether, move with it to reduce the blow.

consistency

Your neighborhood gym's business model relies on this principle being broken. If every member of every gym actually went on a regular basis, you'd always be waiting your turn for equipment or paying much more for a membership.

There are a lot of reasons for missing a workout:

- body is sore
- slept in late or early morning appointment
- after work outing
- ate poorly the meal before workout time, feeling sluggish

I won't discount any of them: life happens. But the good news is we only have to rip 2 workouts per week. So unless you're partying every day or attend breakfast meetings for a living, there is no excuse to not hit your workouts.

If we break up every day into 2 periods, morning and evening, you have 14 "shots" per week to work out. Only 2 of them need to agree with your mood, routine, and schedule. So a 14% conversion rate == 100% success. The odds are in your favor.

If you balk at this, ask yourself: how many of those 14 periods do you find a way to watch Netflix? read hackernews? reddit? Twitter? Facebook? Instagram?

There's no need to berate you on consistency, as fitting our new lifestyle into our old one has been paramount since Chapter 1 of this book. If you can't hack this, you'll never achieve your health goals. Before closing this book, I'd like you to think of a friend you can lend it to, someone who really wants it.

seeing results

Similar to overeating, this, too, has already been solved by multi-dimensional tracking. Instead of looking at our weight alone, we're also measuring muscle size, body fat, composition, and even advanced properties like ketones.

While writing this chapter, I spent a week in Malaysia, speaking at 3 corporate workshops and going out for big meals afterward. I had my first alcoholic beverage in over 2 months. That one drink led to 9 more... it was a 9-course tasting menu, paired with cocktails. I also had some chocolate and sugar. And cake! (*it was my birthday, and the organizer figured it out because processing my invoice required I show them my ID*)

The only areas in which I did not budge during this hell of a week: workouts, fasting, and avoiding bread and rice. Even then, I gained weight. About 8 pounds in 14 days.

Meanwhile, I was still tracking 2-3 gains per week in my fitness regimen. My body—thank you weekly progress pics—looked better too. I was observing bigger arms (my goal) and ever more visible abdomen muscles.

If I was like most people or even my former self, this temporary weight gain might have killed my motivation. That's why we're learning not to rely on motivation alone, but to rely on the aggregate of our metrics, the facts. See, those 8 pounds I gained was primarily water weight, not fat. Within 48 hours of my 9-course meal, I purged nearly all the excess and was back on track.

The bottom line is: sometimes, your scale will disagree with your effort. Some weeks you'll lose (fat) or gain (muscle) effortlessly, and swear your scale is broken. Other times, it will feel like there's a conspiracy against you. There is.

FIRST PRINCIPLES

Treat the previous section like a glossary or 24/7 hotline when you're *jonesin'* to make a mistake. Yes, this is the first time I've ever written "jonesin'" in my entire life.

You might wonder why I haven't spent more pages discussing "hacks" to correct our wrongs. Why haven't I included email scripts you can copy/paste to your boss to skip the next company party? Or some magic pill that will purge you after a night out? (*this pill, by the way, is called Dulcolax.*)

Peter Drucker's *The Effective Executive* warns against this temptation.[4]

He argues that knowledge workers, when faced with decisions, must first determine whether the situation is unique. If the circumstances *are* unique, apply a unique treatment. But if the circumstances have been faced before, apply principles instead.

Drucker describes the four possible categories every decision fits into:

1. recurring; you've seen it before → principles
2. rare; you've never seen it before but others have → principles
3. rare; you've never seen it before but it will soon become normal → principles
4. unique; you've never seen it, neither has anyone else and unlikely to happen again

With all the free, accessible knowledge on dieting, health, and fitness, I'm going to take a leap and assume your situation is not unique and has been dealt with many times before you.

While researching for this book, the most unique circumstance I encountered was from a software engineer in Delhi, India. His challenge is the "quality of air," literally. His enjoyment for cardio and running is squashed on high-pollution days, and this is a very real problem.

Yet even in this case, a few things to consider: the population of Delhi is over 19 million; gyms have treadmills; cardio is a poor way to gain muscle (which is his goal). Whether your town is polluted, green, rural, suburban, or urban, it's likely all your "challenges" can be addressed with principles and alternatives.

DIFFERENT TYPES OF PAIN

As you adopt Fitness for Hackers into your lifestyle, you will discover something: either the dieting is easier, or the workouts are easier. This makes sense because they're different types of pain.

Dieting is marked by *avoidance*. We have to restrict ourselves from kryptonite ingredients that disagree with our metabolism. And even if we can manage this at mealtime, we then have to go hours straight without stuffing our faces after dinner on the couch.

Exercise is marked by *non-avoidance*. We have to confront things. First, by actually going to the gym. Then, by pushing ourselves to finish a rep. And don't stop there, we must finish our set. If we fall short of our set, we have to do an *interest rep* (Chapter 6). And finally, we have to muster the courage to *increase* our number of repetitions or resistance through self-awareness that the discomfort we feel from a given lift is not enough.

In this way, dieting and exercise feel incongruent. And it's probably why we see a lot of "meat heads" with big arms who, frankly, are kind of fat. It's probably why we see models who are "skinny fat" and unable to lift a 5lb dumbbell.

Fitness for Hackers alumni (can I call you that?) accept that there is little compatibility between the mental faculties required to *simultaneously* eat right and lift weights. Then they do both anyway.

Those 10 seconds of extreme muscle stress at the gym represent your body getting stronger. Those 4 hours of fake hunger pangs after dinner, before bed, represent your body getting leaner. You cannot compromise one with the other. But you can acknowledge that one type of pain will likely be easier to manage.

NOTES ON HUNGER

I've alluded to this topic a few times, so let's address it head on: if your new regiment leaves you "always hungry," you are doing it wrong.

I've personally been crushing BBQ, steaks, burgers (no bun), skewers, grilled veggies, and coffee (+ cream OK) for 3 months, and my body is in the greatest shape it's ever been. This diet is heavy on protein and fiber, so it fills you up for longer. We'll review my exact diet in Chapter 9.

Contrast this to previous fitness kicks in my life where I restricted my eating further, worked out 2x as many hours per week, and tried different "hacks' to get out of company parties: Fitness for Hackers is sustainable, kicks are not.

A few thoughts on why you might feel hungry and what to do about it:

- *you're mentally underwhelmed with the volume of food you eat.* If you're like me and enjoy pork, know this 2x as fatty and caloric as steak. If you prefer the visual stimulus of a "large" meal, chicken is leaner, and you can eat a lot more of it with the same outcomes. It's possible you subconsciously seek a certain amount of chewing and aren't really "hungry" at all.
- *you're eating at suboptimal times.* Besides the metabolic benefits of intermittent fasting, it also forces us to be more aware of our needs for sustenance. If, for example, you eat a 300-500 calorie breakfast every day simply because that's what you've always done, you're now limited to a ~1100-1300 appetite for the rest of the day. If that breakfast didn't give you the same boost of energy you get from, say, lunch, you've now fallen prey to diminishing returns, and real hunger later in the day won't be addressed unless you overeat.

- *you're procrastinating.* If a project at work or your front lawn grass needs to be cut, you might use food as an "escape" from responsibility. After all, it takes a few minutes to prepare food, then eat it, then clean up after yourself. If what you crave is 20 minutes away, even better! Be conscientious of when this is happening and question whether you're really hungry, or just being a lazy bum.

DAMAGE CONTROL

I don't endorse this strategy, but I'll tell you what I've done once in the past 3 months to mitigate the damage from a night out of drinking: cleanse. Specifically, I did this after the Malaysia debacle where I gained 8 pounds over a 2 week period of bad choices.

At nearly any local drug or supplement store, you can get a fruity flavored (see: disgusting) bottle of magic juice that will compel a few extra bowel movements within 24 hours. I did this, and the result was a 4-5 pound weight loss in under 2 days. Granted, this was probably mostly water, but it helped me psychologically.

If you're tempted to get a "quick win" from a cleanse, I won't hold it against you. But cleanses are not a sustainable way to lose weight, and sustainability is our aim. Cleanses are also logistically challenging since you pretty much have to run to the bathroom once nature calls. I suggest staying home from work, or cleansing on a weekend if you choose to run this experiment. Godspeed.

GROWTH IS NON-LINEAR

This book could be summarized by the heading above.

As hackers, we are well versed in product iterations, marketing campaign iterations, organizational, and structural iterations. With each tweak made to the system, the system improves.

But that's not always true, is it? This assumes every decision we make is correct. And it further assumes that the market—something external and out of our control—will respond to our rationality in-kind.

Sadly, this isn't how it works. In a fitness context, our body is, to some degree, like the market. We don't totally understand it. We pitch (feed) it things, and then it reacts. We provide it the tools we've determined will make it successful (strength training), then it reacts.

Just as business growth is non-linear, so is our personal fitness. And we can tell ourselves this over and again, but it won't be internalized until you have a moment like I did, stepping on a scale in Cambodia last week, 8 pounds fatter because of a few poor choices I made in Malaysia.

The best way to prepare your mind for non-linear growth is to recall that we are not beholden to a single variable. Sure, you might gain a few pounds. But how's your energy level? Are your pants loose around the waist? Do you still get compliments at work?

The audacity for an entrepreneur to assume they will never have a down month (lower revenue than the period before) is always challenged after enough years in business. At my own company, Fomo, we grew 19 months straight before our first down month. When it happened, I laid in bed for 2 days and started watching *This Is Us*.

So embrace the suck. Accept now, in Week 1 or 2 of your journey, that you won't always step on the scale and see the results you've modeled. Sometimes you'll feel like you're moving backward. And when that happens, realize the only way out is *through*.[5]

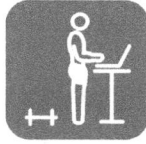

CHAPTER 8

ADVANCED TECHNIQUES TO 10X YOUR PROGRESS

"People always tell you, 'Be humble. Be humble.' When was the last time someone told you to be amazing? Be great! Be great! Be awesome! Be awesome!"
— Kanye West

Many readers will see results in just a week or two. If you don't "see" them, you'll feel it. But like all challenges in life, once we get the hang of something, it tends to get boring.

A few weeks ago, my wife booked us 3 games of laser tag at a place well known for corporate outings, aka adult players. Well, only 12-year-old German kids showed up, and it was a bloodbath. I was Umbriel.

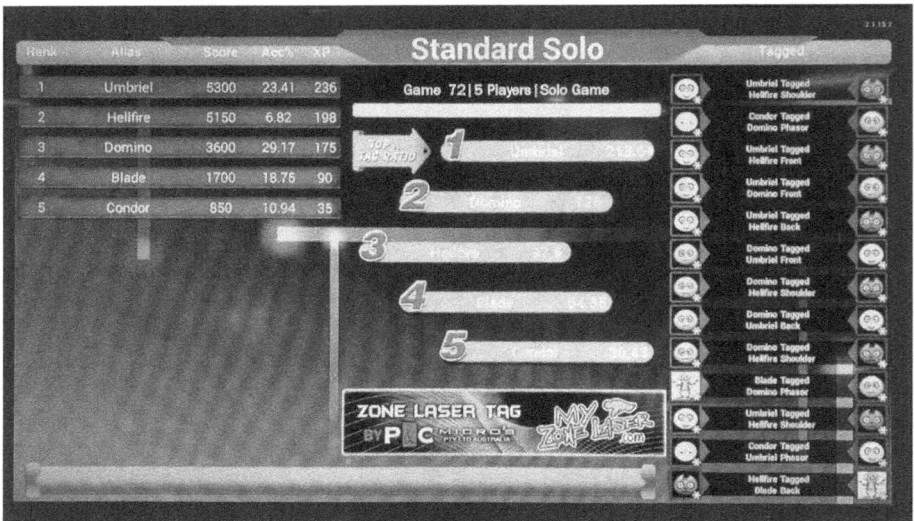

While the win might have stroked my ego, it didn't make me much better at laser tag to compete against preteen boys. Doing the same number of repetitions at the same weight will also get easier over time, but it doesn't make us ripped.

The central premise of a personal trainer is to push you further than you'd push yourself. We can save thousands of dollars per year by being our own personal trainer. To do this effectively, we'll use a system called *gain velocity*.

GAIN VELOCITY

In software development, it's a well-known joke that estimating how long it will take to do something is a nearly impossible task. For this reason, developers have invented terminology to grasp progress, terms like velocity, volume, t-shirt size, and so on.

Velocity is how often a team finishes tasks, small or large. *Volume* is the number of tasks completed in a given time period. *T-Shirt size* is used to estimate the complexity of a given task, which usually means it will take longer to complete.

The idea behind each of these terms is that a manager, especially those who aren't technical, can still judge the performance of their team without using misleading metrics like lines of code.

A similar notion exists in film. A director friend once told me:

> *"you spend 90% of your time on the first 90% of the movie, then 90% of your time on the last 10% of the movie."*

Because we know fitness growth is non-linear, we need a yardstick with which to measure progress that incorporates estimation futility. We need to be able to parse our historical progress—even on a "fat day" where we weigh 8 pounds more than last week—with a lens that reflects its environment.

To set this up, let's refer to our Trello board, which is already tracking resistance gains.

If you're a few weeks into your 90-day fitness experiment, you have some sense of gain velocity already: how many Trello "cards" are you moving to your Gains list on a weekly basis?

This can be simplified as how many gains you accumulate per workout. In my own regimen, I see 1-3 gains per week, for an average of 2 gains per week, or 1 gain per gym session.

Calculate your own GPW (gains per workout) and revisit monthly to evaluate if your velocity is consistent. If it is, great. If it isn't, you're not being a very good personal trainer.

Disclaimer: it's natural to track a lot more gains in the early weeks of your program simply because your body is going "Zero to One." The novelty alone might spur additional energy reserves, and it's also likely you underestimated yourself in setting up inaugural lift metrics (Chapter 4).

That said, you should not be content with a plateau unless you're in maintenance mode. We'll discuss this in the last chapter because it implies you've achieved your fitness goals. At this point, though, you haven't.

BENCHMARKING THE BENCHMARKS

In Chapter 4 we kick-started our fitness experiment with a handful of lifts. Each one was accompanied with a repetition count and appropriately paired resistance (weight) level for our body.

Then we started lifting, experiencing gains, and… arbitrarily determining the new number of repetitions or resistance to conquer in our next iteration of that lift.

As an example, progress over time for bicep curls might look like this:

- Week 1 - 50lbs, 7 repetitions
- Week 2 - 50lbs, 11 repetitions
- Week 3 - 55lbs, 8 repetitions
- Week 4 - 60lbs, 4 repetitions

If we're not careful, we may be playing a game of "fudge the numbers" as we resort to higher resistance and lower repetitions every time we think we're due a gain.

To end this guessing game (insanity) let's introduce another system: 6-8-10.

6-8-10 GAINS

Instead of flipping a coin and asking if you should increase resistance *or* increase repetitions count, this process will help you do both systematically. The "how" is baked right into the name.

For each of your lifts, starting with the ones where you've plateaued, reset your resistance to whatever amount of weight you can do for *6 straight repetitions*. In upcoming workouts, don't mark a gain until you can do 8 straight repetitions, then 10 straight repetitions.

You'll probably have 1-2 workout sessions where you can do 7, or 9. The in-between numbers. Definitely do these reps, but don't clock it as a gain.

Once you hit 10 reps, consider this lift "baked." increase your resistance by 2, 5, or 10 pounds, then restart at 6 repetitions. Repeat this metric refactoring for each of your lifts.

If you're applying 6-8-10 and still hitting plateaus, simply reorder your lifts. Drag and drop your Trello cards to put the most challenging, stubborn lift first in your session. I've observed that compound lifts like squats require more reserved energy than biceps, so doing squats first thing keeps me explosive.

PRESENCE AND MEDITATION AT THE GYM

By implementing 6-8-10 a few things happen:

- plateaus don't last as long
- gym time does not require an active brain
- workouts are easier to memorize

Some readers in my "beta tester" audience griped to me that their biggest challenge with workouts is having the mental energy to do it. Some of our jobs are incredibly demanding on our creative and computational skills, and once we're done for the day, we're *done* in every sense of the word.

I did not address this in Troubleshooting (Chapter 7) for two reasons. First, terms like "burned out" and "exhausted" are highly subjective. As we recall about a personal trainer's ability to push us further than we push ourselves, there's a suspicious sentiment about exhaustion in that it's always expressed by the exhausted, never by their observer.

If your wife or roommate says, "you don't talk to me after work, you're always so exhausted," then you have some evidence. But if all the complaining is from your mouth alone, I call BS.

The second reason I did not address mental exhaustion or burnout in Troubleshooting is because the 6-8-10 system helps alleviate it. Eckhart Tolle's explosive bestseller *The Power of Now* describes[6] what happens when we focus on what we're doing right now, vs. allowing our minds to wander and compute the future or past. Paraphrased:

> "being in a state of no-mind does not mean you aren't able to think… it means you choose to think and treat your mind (brain) as a tool to be picked up and put back down again…"

By eliminating variables in your fitness routine, you give your brain a chance to rest even while your body is working harder than ever.

When you extend this variable elimination practice into other areas of your regimen, e.g. living close to a gym, patronizing one with showers to reduce logistical challenges, scheduling meals, or workouts ahead of time… you again increase the energy reserves to achieve your fitness goals, despite "exhaustion" from your day job.

COMPETE WITH YOURSELF

This is for ambitious readers only. After nailing your workout routine, monitoring gain velocity over time, and getting past the social humps of saying "no" (diet) and saying "yes" (exercise), you'll again ask yourself: now what?

The answer to that question is a return to a concept introduced in Chapter 2—*via negativa*.

Identify one part of your lifestyle that, if eliminated, would lead to better health. For me, this was going out with my single friends, and to eliminate them, I ended my apartment lease and booked a 1-way ticket across the planet.

If that's too extreme for you, I understand. Try the following instead:

- stay home 1 weekend per month (or two, or three…)
- stop eating _____ (for me this is milk; in non-linear fitness periods I eliminate milk to simplify variables)
- make public commitments

Let's explore the last one because I find this to be the most difficult for the average Joe.

There's a saying that on social networks like Twitter, 99% of users are consumers, and only 1% create. I'm not sure how factual this is, but the sentiment remains: most people are private.

This is OK ethically, legally, spiritually. But being private about your fitness goals can put them at risk, as it robs you of the endless benefits of *accountability*.

ACCOUNTABILITY IS A FAT-BURNING MACHINE

Blogger Thomas Oppong wrote an excellent piece on the topic of accountability, premised on the following insight from The American Society of Training and Development:

> *[ASTD] did a study on accountability and found that you have a 65% chance of completing a goal if you commit to someone. And if you have a specific accountability appointment with a person you've committed, you will increase your chance of success by up to 95%.*[7]

This is almost hard to believe. A 95% chance of success is almost like saying you'll get a brain transplant and occupy the body of a wholly different person, simply by telling someone what you intend to do.

In my pre-launch book audience, I asked for a similar commitment in exchange for early access to these chapters. What's your current weight? what's your goal weight? You better believe I'm following up with all the readers who provided these figures.

If you agree the benefits of accountability outweigh the costs a small dent in privacy, here's something you can do. It's a classic move by this author, as all I can offer are things I've done myself: Tweet.

I don't care if you have 5 followers or 500, Tweet that you're working on getting in shape. That you intend to lose X or gain Y, that your body fat is currently Z, but you want it to be XYZ. Just make a public commitment and see what happens.

This goes beyond fitness, by the way. I can't even count how many times I've used this trick to achieve all sorts of things:

- "tonight I'm publishing a blog post about _____"
- "next week I'm launching a new app on Product Hunt"
- "by this summer I'll be ripped"
- "writing a book about how to stay in shape as a hacker…"

Leverage the power of self-fulfilling prophecy through public accountability. If Tweeting specifically isn't your thing, apps like SPAR![8] let you remain some-what private within the confines of their community while also putting real money on the line. If you commit to a task and don't complete it regularly, you have to pay. And if you stick to your habits, you get paid. It's neat.

Long before I pieced together the Fitness for Hackers philosophy, some col-leagues at my coworking space in San Francisco arrived at the same conclusion: every day we were to meet on the roof and do as many pushups as we could in 3 minutes.

Unable to help myself, I built www.pushupmetrics.com in 48 hours while visiting my parents for Christmas break.

Within a week, we had multi-tenancy, which meant we could all join the "team" for our coworking space and compare stats. In the following months, we extended the app to include SMS alerts at 2:55p. My final feature, when I knew I'd gone too far, was integrating a weather API that instructed everyone to go to the basement instead of the roof if it was raining.

I've since sold this app to another entrepreneur, but you can still sign up to log your pushups or compete with friends and colleagues.

PERSEVERANCE

I'd be remiss if I didn't write this word at least once.

One of my business ventures is an online marketing course, and occasionally a thief will attempt to steal the content and resell it on their own website. Usually, these charges are blocked by my payment processor, but one time a thief managed to enroll at full price ($2,100 USD) and access my lectures.

Shortly after, they filed an "item not delivered" chargeback claim. I appealed, providing ample evidence as well as proof my material was stolen and being resold. This claim was denied, and $2,100 was deducted from my bank account. Ouch.

Luckily I was able to "appeal the appeal," and in doing so I won the case, reverting the $2,100 back into my possession. Next, I got my course removed from the illegal website. And to top it all off, I wrote a recap that was quickly featured on the homepage of BoingBoing, Digg, and other prominent websites, driving thousands of readers to my website and 100s of comments.

In retelling this story on my blog, I synthesized a single piece of advice relevant to our fitness routine: *"entrepreneurs aren't just people who keep trying. They are the ones who keep trying until it works."*

As you modify lifts, reps, diet restrictions, and personal schedules to accommodate the Fitness for Hackers regimen, remove all caps. By 'cap' I mean arbitrary limits dictating *when* something should work. Our new mindset requires us to keep trying *until* it works.

Put another way, just remember Newton's first law: a gym-goer in motion stays in motion.

INCREASE THE DIFFICULTY

If your workout routine is baked into your lifestyle, you've eliminated calorie-excessive habits to accelerate growth, and gains are predictable with the 6-8-10 system, you're ready for a final challenge: More.

Throughout this book, I've stressed a twice per week, 25 minutes per session, workout experiment. And indeed, for the first 10 weeks of this program, I personally followed it to the dot.

But now, on Week 13, as I write this section, my body is hungry for *more*. So I've increased my regimen from 2 workouts per week to 3. I also added a C-Day to my Trello board, which has new workouts involving my abdomen muscle groups.

This one tweak let me exploit my body's natural longing for more discipline, as well as mitigates my otherwise sluggish growth on workouts like squats and deadlifts. When you introduce a new muscle group to your regimen, the entire experiment starts over, as each group complements the others.

Aesthetic gaps are also easily addressed with a 3rd workout or C-Day implementation. For me, I was happy seeing my arms get bigger, and my waist get smaller, but I still had visible "love handles" and was not enjoying abs, even at 9.5% body fat (see my InBody results in Chapter 4).

My C-Day incorporates torso curls, crunches, and decline weighted sit-ups to fill this void, which was not covered directly in the base level Fitness for Hackers regimen.

To capture more value from Fitness for Hackers after your initial goals are reached, simply increase the difficulty and start the clock over again.

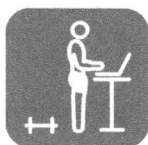

CHAPTER 9

MAINTENANCE AND LONG-TERM GOALS

*"The final forming of a person's character
lies in their own hands."*
— Anne Frank

If your goal is to lose 5 or 10 pounds, or even 20, you'll probably achieve it by the end of our 90-day experiment. At this point, you have to decide: set a new goal or switch to maintenance mode?

The previous chapter shared a few techniques to level up your regimen for new goals. In this chapter, we'll discuss how to keep what you've earned.

DIET NORMALIZATION

If your favorite foods are off-diet, 3 months is a long time to go without them. Living in NYC made pizza and FroYo (frozen yogurt) a near staple in my routine, for example. But when I finally got serious about my health, I stopped eating both.

It's true what they say: a cheat meal won't kill you. But it will make you feel fat for a day, and possibly reflect itself disproportionately on the scale, should you check the next morning.

For those in maintenance mode, get comfortable with this tradeoff. Have 1 cheat meal per week so you can stop losing your mind, then be a good boy come Monday lest you digress back to your old ways.

EXERCISE NORMALIZATION

In following the 6-8-10 lift sequence, take as long as you need to max out each of your repetition <> resistance combinations until you're doing 10 repetitions per lift. Then, stop calculating gains.

Unlike dieting, which is the primary source of weight loss, we can't simply do "more" or "less" exercise to dramatically change our body mass. But you can stop endeavoring to achieve your measured gain velocity, and you can cut your workouts from 3x /week (if you followed the 10x rule) to just twice per week, 25 minutes per session.

To be clear: exercise will never go away. If you interpret maintenance mode to "stop working out," you will get fat again, and it will be all your fault.

Accept that being healthy means exercising on a weekly basis for the rest of your life. There is no shortcut here. This is again why I recommend "fancy" gyms if you can afford it. You will be spending a lot of time at the gym. Invest in yourself.

DIET REDUX

I left you hanging a bit on the topic of food. It's possible you've been restricting yourself beyond what's necessary. Because I'm not a nutritionist, I can't prescribe exactly what to eat, but I can share what I eat on any given week.

Here are a few of my most recent meals, taken from my calorie tracker app:

- Lunch - 2 chicken breast skewers, 1 pork tenderloin skewer, 1 bag of pork rinds

- Dinner - Korean BBQ (skirt steak, duck breast, pork belly, kimchi, miso paste, onions, salad)
- Lunch - grilled chicken caesar salad with bacon and egg, tomato bisque soup
- Dinner - triple grilled cheeseburger with bacon, lettuce, tomato (no bun)
- Lunch - cold cuts from the grocery store (prosciutto, sharp cheddar cheese, pepperoni, black forest ham)
- Dinner - tandoori chicken, garlic chicken, chana masala
- Lunch - grilled pork chop and asparagus
- Dinner - mixed fajitas (steak, chicken, shrimp), no tortillas or rice

I usually eat 500-700 calories for lunch and 800-1200 calories for dinner. I'm able to do this because I skip breakfast (fasting). And I curb my "snack" appetite in two ways. First, my feeding window is just 6-8 hours. I don't need more than 2 meals in such a short period. Second, coffee.

COFFEE IS A DIETING TOOL

Coffee (caffeine) helps us focus, stay alert, and just plain get through the workday as a social gathering mechanism. It also has chlorogenic acids, a kind of antioxidant that some scientists believe suppresses your appetite.

Experimental results are mixed, but if it works for you, it works.[9]

When I drink coffee on an empty stomach, say in the morning while I'm fasting before lunch, it gives my stomach a bit of a slap in the face. At first, this felt like nausea, now I think of it as a metabolic juice, revving up my calorie-burning engine for the day's first meal.

In the evening, I also drink coffee, not only to stay alert and work after dinner but also to give my hands and mouth something to *do*. There's a lot of compelling evidence that smokers who try to quit, but fail, are perhaps not so much addicted to the nicotine as they are the ritual of engaging their hands and mouth, known as oral fixation.[10]

CLIMBING VS. HANGING

When you're dieting and working out according to this book's recommendation, your intensity level on a 1-10 scale is a 7. If you take advantage of the 10x techniques in Chapter 8, this might be an 8. Let's reserve the 9-10 cohort for professional athletes and bodybuilders who train for hours every day.

We know that achieving our fitness goals is a bit of a paradox in that we are practicing avoidance (dieting) and non-avoidance (exercise) simultaneously. The crux of maintenance mode, then, is successfully toggling between the two states.

In doing so, fitness becomes a background job in our lifestyle instead of feeling like the center of it. If you're reading or re-reading this section after a few weeks on the program, you can probably attest to this.

Starting out can feel like our life has been taken over by a bunch of new rules—eat this, do that, resist some other thing. But as we bend fitness to our will, and not the other way around, health is no more mentally exhausting than making our bed.

LONG-TERM GOALS

Maybe "lose 5 more pounds" or "reduce body fat 1%" isn't exciting to you after achieving your initial goals.

For married readers, especially, this is sensible. You don't have to attract a mate, you aren't a professional athlete whose income depends on your fitness, and nothing is looming around the corner that demands a peek health state.

But what if there was?

I've observed countless friends commit as far as 12 months in advance to run marathons or compete in a Spartan, Tough Mudder, or Iron Man race. Not to "win," but to give themselves a specific reason for maintaining a level of fitness. Also, because it's fun.

My first half marathon was a few years ago in Brooklyn. My max distance during training was 7 miles, so I wasn't sure how my body would fare running nearly double that on race day. Then it happened, and I got literal chills as thousands of people cheered us on from the sidelines. The entire race was kind of a blur and nothing like training. I ran 2 more races in the next 12 months.

If you don't want to pin a new metric to set the bar higher for yourself, commit to a public event that will force you to maintain what you already earned. The experience will be unforgettable, and you deserve to be proud of yourself.

TAKE PHOTOS

Throughout the fitness experiment, you should have been taking progress pics. This makes it easier to objectively measure improvements over time when the mirror doesn't make it obviously clear.

But even now, while you're past the finish line, you should keep taking photos for the reverse effect: to know if you're regressing.

I don't expect you to keep calorie counting after the 90-day mark, because whatever you eat for a quarter of a year is probably what you'll eat for the next quarter of the year. When you cut off all the tracking mechanisms, however, it does make you more liable to slip. To snacking.

So, keep taking photos. You don't need to be naked. Social memories with friends will suffice. And if those pictures start to bother you, re-read this book. Your mindset got lost, so let's find it again first, then get back in the gym.

Another reason to take photos: it's possible you picked up this book because you didn't like how you looked in a recent photo. Pictures, then, are a great litmus test for measuring our perceived health. Fancy apps and spreadsheets aside, take and *look* at photos of yourself to catch leading indicators of regression.

PART III NOTES

1. Mark Manson, If Self-Discipline Feels Difficult, Then You're Doing it Wrong, Feb 8, 2019
2. James Clear, Atomic Habits, The Four Laws of Behavior Change, Chapter 3
3. USDA FoodData Central, https://fdc.nal.usda.gov/fdc-app.html#/, query "alcoholic"
4. Peter Drucker, The Effective Executive
5. Robert Frost, A Servant to Servants, 1915
6. Eckhart Tolle, Power of Now
7. Thomas Oppong, "This is How to Increase the Odds of Reaching your Goals by 95%" citing The American Society of Training and Development (ASTD), https://medium.com/the-mission/the-accountability-effect-a-simple-way-to-achieve-your-goals-and-boost-your-performance-8a07c76ef53a
8. SPAR!, https://getspar.com
9. "Coffee and appetite: Does coffee make you more or less hungry?", https://www.precisionnutrition.com/research-review-coffee-hunger
10. "Chew On This: The Need to Engage Your Mouth and Hands After Quitting", https://www.quitterscircle.com/staying-smokefree/chew-on-this-the-need-to-engage-your-mouth-and-hands-after-quitting

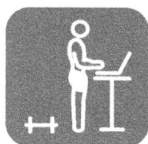

CONCLUSION

Welcome to the end. Perhaps you read this book in one sitting. Enlightened readers will recognize a few missing pieces:

- there is no discussion on "stretching"
- there is no discussion on "drinking lots of water"
- there is little discussion of nutrition and biology

These gaps are intentional. Reading between the lines of prose, Fitness for Hackers is a book about mindset as much as it is about fitness.

You see, before penning the first chapter. I knew a few things about forthcoming readers:

- you've already read a fitness book (or two, or three)
- you've already tried to get in shape, then relapsed

One 'aha' moment in my own life, irrespective of health and wellness and technology, is the distinction between "simple" and "easy." While many texts promise the latter, they muddy the former.

Fitness for Hackers outlines a simple, but not easy, approach to getting in the best shape of your life. It explains how to do so with minimal time investment (easy) and rigid principles (simple).

Adopting a new diet and exercise routine is like learning any other skill; it becomes easier after getting over the learning curve. We can identify the learning curve as inertia, and identify the motivation from seeing results as habit-forming momentum.

At the risk of upsetting my publisher, I'll go a step further and confess something: I *hope* your reaction to this book is "*that's it?*" because yes, that is it.

A lot of would-be entrepreneurs get stuck in the Do Nothing Loop. It looks like this: think about starting a company, research how to start a company, learn about successful companies, do nothing about it, then restart.

People who are out of shape act the same way about fitness. They obsess over the science, seeking premature optimizations. But just like choosing your first programming language, the most important thing is to *just start*. You will modify your plan (diet + exercise routine) as you progress.

Here are this book's key points:

- you can do anything (Part 1)
- what gets measured, gets managed (Part 2)
- sustainability is a function of habits (Part 3)

Now that you have the tools, it's time to go lift weight. To network with other readers, visit fitnessforhackers.com.

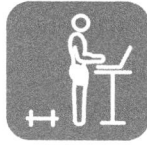

SHOWING MY WORK

I implemented this book's ideas before I wrote them. Everything I've suggested was tested on my own body before I recommended it for yours.

Here are my results from 90 days of dieting, working out 2x /week, then 3x for the last couple weeks, intermittent fasting, and tracking everything in Zero, MyFitnessPal, and a Spreadsheet.

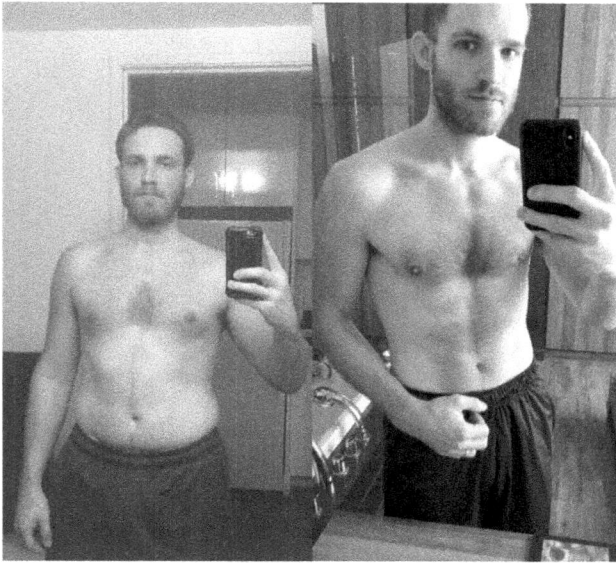

Oh, and I did it all while traveling full-time in 8 countries and 10 cities:

- 26.6 pounds lost (196 → 169.4)
- 51 gains (velocity of 4.25 per week, or 2.125 per session)

- 1.5 inch reduction in leg circumference
- 2.5 inches reduce in waist circumference (in other words, down 2 pants sizes)
- 1.25 inch increase in bicep circumference
- visible abdomen muscles

My next goal is to improve my abs to 6- or 8-pack status. To achieve this, I've made my 3rd weekly workout, or C-Day, all about core. You know, the stuff that makes you want to throw up: crunches, sit-ups, planks.

I didn't write this book to make money, I wrote it to make hackers fit. If you bought this book from my website, send me your before/after progress pics for a refund: progress@fitnessforhackers.com.

The world needs you to build the future. Your family needs you to exist. And you need the best tool to do it with: you.

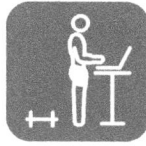

SPECIAL THANKS

Adil Majid
Amrik Deol
Andrew Byers
Binh Wilson
Cameron Smith
Cameron Wiese
Candace Wu
Gabriel Rotaru
Giovanni Luperti
Joshua Dance
Kameron Kales
Kyle Duck
Kyle Tan
Manuel Frigerio
Mike Rubini
Mike Smith
Shane Forrester
Trevor Sookraj
Val Pinkhasov
Will McLellarn

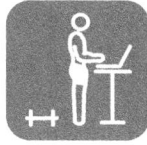

GLOSSARY

6-8-10 - process of increasing set repetitions and weight by incrementing reps from 6 to 10, then weight, then restarting

conspiracy against your health - mental model for understanding why bad foods are cheap, free, and highly accessible

gain velocity - lift improvements over time, measured as the average # of improvements per workout session

gym anxiety - the phenomenon that people are watching or judging you at the gym; they are not, they don't care about

interest repetition - a single repetition, in addition to your documented set expectation, required when you cannot complete a set of repetitions in one motion

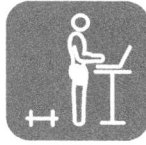

BIO

Ryan Kulp is a founder, marketer, and developer. He's worked with dozens of venture-backed companies on product and marketing strategy and written hundreds of essays on growth and leadership at ryanckulp.com.

Currently, Ryan is leading Fomo.com "in the open" (fomo.com/open) and acquiring small software companies with his wife at Fork Equity (forkequity.com).

Ryan grew up in Atlanta and lives between New York City, San Francisco, and Texas. In 2019 Ryan began a trip around the world and is documenting the experience at rickshawlabs.com.

www.ingramcontent.com/pod-product-compliance
Lightning Source LLC
Chambersburg PA
CBHW050124280326
41933CB00010B/1230